J. F. Debatin   G. C. McKinnon

Ultrafast MRI

Springer

Berlin
Heidelberg
New York
Barcelona
Budapest
Hongkong
London
Milan
Paris
Santa Clara
Singapore
Tokyo

J. F. Debatin   G. C. McKinnon

Ultrafast MRI

Techniques and Applications

With Contributions by
I. Berry, J.F. Debatin, J. Doornbos, P. Duthil,
S. Göhde, H.J. Lamb, G.C. McKinnon, D.A. Leung,
J.-P. Ranjeva, C. Manelfe, A. de Roos

With 295 Figures

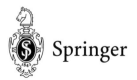 Springer

Debatin, Jörg F., MD
Institute of Diagnostic Radiology
University Hospital Zürich
Rämistrasse 100, CH-8091 Zürich
Switzerland

McKinnon, Graeme C., PhD
GE Medical Systems
PO Box 414, W-875
Milwaukee, WI 53201
USA

ISBN 3-540-62765-0 Springer-Verlag Berlin Heidelberg New York

Library of Congress Cataloging-in-Publication Data

Ultrafast MRI: techniques and applications/ [edited by] Jörg F. Debatin,
Graeme C. McKinnon; with contributions by I. Berry [et al.].
    p.   cm.
Includes bibliographical references and index.
ISBN 3-540-62765-0 (hardcover)
1. Magnetic resonance. I. Debatin, Jörg F., 1961– II. McKinnon, Graeme C.
(Graeme Colin), 1955– III. Berry, I. (Isabelle)
[DNLM: 1. Magnetic Resonance Imaging – method.   WN 185 U47 1998]
RC78.7.N83U48   1998
616.07'548 – dc21
DNLM/DLC
for Library of Congress   97-40499
                                                CIP

Cover: E. Kirchner
Typesetting: Michael Kusche, Goldener Schnitt

SPIN: 10748969   21/3111 – 5 4 3 2 1 – Printed on acid-free paper

Contents

2   Ultrafast Magnetic Resonance Imaging of the Brain and Spine

I. BERRY, J.-P. RANJEVA, P. DUTHIL, C. MANELFE

3   Ultrafast Magnetic Resonance Imaging of the Heart

H.J. LAMB, J. DOORNBOS, A. DE ROOS

**4   Ultrafast Magnetic Resonance Imaging
        of the Vascular System**
        D.A. LEUNG, J.F. DEBATIN

5 Ultrafast Magnetic Resonance Imaging of the Abdomen
S.C. GÖHDE, J.F. DEBATIN

Preface

The imaging potential of the MR experiment continues to evolve. In recent years, an increasing number of fast and ultrafast imaging strategies has been described. In this evolution the definition of the terms fast and ultrafast has been blurred. Hence they are frequently used interchangeably. The evolution of these methods has been based on two related, yet separate developments: an increasingly thorough understanding of the complexities inherent to pulse sequence design and the increasing availability of stronger and faster gradient systems. The combination of these two factors has laid the foundation for vast reductions of MRI data acquisition times. Minutes have been replaced by seconds. Beyond shortening MR examination times and thereby increasing patient throughput, a most significant consequence has been the ability to acquire complex MR image sets within the time confines of a single breath-hold. The constraints placed by the presence of respiratory motion have thus been effectively eliminated. Ultrafast breath-held data acquisition strategies already represent the backbone of many abdominal, thoracic and even pelvic imaging protocols. The enhanced image quality permits full exploitation of the unsurpassed soft tissue contrast inherent to the MR experiment. Beyond improving the quality of existing applications, the implementation of ultrafast imaging techniques has permitted the exploration of new imaging indications, particularly in the area of perfusion and diffusion as well as ultrafast 3D imaging.

The success of fast and ultrafast imaging techniques is reflected by their widespread incorporation into clinical practice in centers throughout the world. They have been applied to various imaging regions, using widely different magnets and data acquisition strategies. As is the case for most MR imaging techniques, a thorough understanding of the underlying mechanisms and proper technique are essential to fully exploit their diagnostic potential.

The book attempts to bridge the gap separating MR scientists into physicists and engineers on one hand and clinicians on the other. It is designed to be of benefit to both groups by describing the technical basis of fast and ultrafast MR imaging and placing these strategies into a clinical context for neurologic, cardiac, vascular, and abdominal imaging applications. These regions were chosen as they appear most significantly impacted by ultrafast MR imaging. All major strategies for fast and ultrafast data collection are discussed in view of potential advantages and disadvantages. Furthermore, various means of accelerating the data collection process are described. The first chapter is rounded off by a concise discussion of hardware requirements. The following four chapters contain a detailed discussion of existent and future applications of fast and ultrafast imaging pertaining to the brain, heart, vessels as well as liver, spleen pancreas and kidneys. Furthermore, the potential of MR colonography and gastrography is high-lighted.

We gratefully acknowledge the contributions by Dr. Isabelle Berry (Chap. 2), and Dr. Albert de Roos (Chap. 3) and their respective coauthors. These experts were successful in providing important insights into their respective fields. We thank Antoinette Schumacher for her diligent review of the manuscripts, and Dr. Susanne Göhde for preparing the index. Furthermore we acknowledge the valuable contributions of Doris Engelhardt at Springer-Verlag and Rainer Kusche, production editor.

November 1997

Jörg F. Debatin, MD
Graeme C. McKinnon, Ph.D

Prologue: How fast is ultrafast?

Defining the exact meaning of "ultrafast" as it pertains to MR imaging is difficult. Although the term is frequently used, all attempts to render a precise definition seem too contrived. For certain techniques, ultrafast means the acquisition of an image in 100 ms or less; for others, it implies completing data collection within the confines of a 30-s breath-hold. Generally, echo-planar, spiral, and fast spin-echo imaging are considered ultrafast; some of the most clinically relevant ultrafast imaging, however, is performed with conventional gradient-recalled-echo sequences. In the end we decided to include all those clinically useful techniques that operate near the technical limits of a modern high-performance MR unit.

List of Contributors

BERRY, ISABELLE, MD PhD
  Department of Neuroradiology,
  University Hospital Purpan,
  Place du Dr Baylac, F-31059 Toulouse Cédex,
  France

DEBATIN, JÖRG F., MD
  Institute of Diagnostic Radiology,
  University Hospital Zürich,
  Rämistrasse 100, CH-8091 Zürich,
  Switzerland

DOORNBOS, JOOST, PhD
  Department of Radiology, Building 1-C2S,
  University Hospital Leiden,
  P.O.Box 9600, 2300 RC Leiden,
  The Netherlands

DUTHIL, PIERRE, PhD
  Department of Biophysics,
  University Hospital Rangueil,
  Avenue Jean Poulhès, 3103 Toulouse Cédex
  France

GÖHDE, SUSANNE C., MD
  Institute of Diagnostic Radiology,
  University Hospital Zürich,
  Rämistrasse 100, CH-8091 Zürich,
  Switzerland

LAMB, HILDO J., MSc
  Department of Radiology, Building 1-C2S,
  University Hospital Leiden,
  P.O.Box 9600, 2300 RC Leiden,
  The Netherlands

LEUNG, DANIEL A., MD
    Institute of Diagnostic Radiology,
    University Hospital Zürich,
    Rämistrasse 100, CH-8091 Zürich,
    Switzerland

MANELFE, CLAUDE, MD
    Department of Neuroradiology,
    University Hospital Purpan,
    Place du Dr Baylac, F-31059 Toulouse Cédex,
    France

MCKINNON, GRAEME C., PHD
    GE Medical Systems,
    PO Box 414, W-875,
    Milwaukee, WI 53201,
    USA

RANJEVA, JEAN-PHILIPPE, PHD
    Department of Neuroradiology ,
    University Hospital Purpan,
    Place du Dr Baylac, F-31059 Toulouse Cédex,
    France

DE ROOS, ALBERT, MD
    Department of Radiology, Building 1-C2S,
    University Hospital Leiden,
    P.O.Box 9600, 2300 RC Leiden,
    The Netherlands

1 The Physics of Ultrafast MRI

G. McKinnon

1 Introduction

The key to understanding magnetic resonance imaging (MRI) is appreciating its vector nature. Most medical imaging modalities deal with scalar quantities. Thus conventional X-rays image absorbtivity, while the ultrasound image is based on reflectivity. The values of scalar attributes can be described by single numbers. Hence it is relatively straightforward to map either of these quantities into a gray scale (or color) image.

With MRI, on the other hand, the situation is somewhat more complex. The quantity being measured, or imaged, is a vector. Thus an object being imaged by MRI appears as a vector distribution. Conceptually this could pose problems with respect to the display of such an object, as vectors are typically represented by arrows. Fortunately, however, quantifying just the scalar length of the vector is sufficient for most MRI applications. Hence the vector nature of MR is not apparent in most clinical MR images. Nevertheless it is central to the imaging process.

Although the nuclear magnetic resonance spin is typically discussed in terms of a three-dimensional (3D) vector, only the components perpendicular to the main magnetic field (the transverse spin components) are important towards understanding the imaging mathematics. These can be described by two-dimensional (2D) vectors. 2D vectors are specified completely by two numbers and a reference frame.

Vectors differ from scalars in, among other things, the manner in which they are added together. Graphically vectors are depicted by arrows with a length and orientation. With MRI these little arrows are imaged, whereby the arrow for a given picture element (pixel) represents the average of all the 2D transverse spin vectors within an image volume element (voxel).

The mathematics describing the image generation process can be considered a notation for describing, firstly, how these transverse spin vectors are rotated by the gradient fields, and, secondly, how a collection of these spin vectors adds up to produce a signal.

Section 2 introduces the spin vector, complex numbers, and a concise notation for vector rotations. It also introduces Fourier transforms and shows how these can be used to describe the summation of transverse spin vectors in the MRI situation. Section 3 reviews the imaging basics of slice selection, phase encoding, frequency encoding, and signal detection. k-Space is introduced in Sect. 4. The k-space description utilizes the previously developed Fourier transform ideas. Also the image signal-to-noise ratio dependencies are derived. The relationship between k-space and certain data acquisition and image reconstruction parameters relevant for fast imaging are covered in Sect. 5. This includes the effects of k-space coverage, the manner in which k-space symmetries can be used to reduce the imaging time, and zero filling as a means of improving the displayed image resolution.

These basics provide a platform upon which fast imaging sequences can be designed. For the design of useful sequences coherent pathways need to be considered. This is described in Sect. 6. Basically, closely spaced radio frequency (RF) pulses set up multiple spin and stimulated echoes, in addition to the free induction decay signal. These all contribute to the measured signal. Image artifacts can easily occur if the phase of these signals is not properly controlled. The steady-state aspects of short TR gradient-echo based sequences are examined in Sect. 7. Currently these remain clinically the most important sequences for ultrafast MRI. In Sect. 8 echo-planar-like imaging sequences are discussed. Conventional echo-planar imaging (EPI), spiral imaging, and the more familiar fast spin-echo (FSE), or RARE, sequences are covered. An important aspect of cardiac and abdominal imaging is dealing with physiological motion. One approach is simply to perform the imaging extremely rapidly. However, for high-resolution imaging physiological gating strategies, as presented in Sect. 9, are useful. Finally, hardware considerations pertaining to ultrafast MRI, including gradient slew rate, gradient amplitude, and sampling bandwidth, are discussed in Sect. 10.

2 Background Theory

In this section the basic mathematical concepts required for understanding the MR experiment are developed. This begins with vectors, introduces the complex number notation for describing them, and then shows how in certain circumstances they can be described by Fourier transforms. The complementary nature of Fourier and real space is illustrated in one and two dimensions.

2.1 The Spin Vector

MRI is concerned with imaging the distribution of nuclear spins. A spin is a vector object. In MRI the spin is a 3D vector. Conventionally a coordinate system is used with the z axis aligned in the direction of the main magnetic field (Fig. 1). In the fully relaxed state the spin vector points along the z axis. When the spin is excited, it precesses about the z axis. In this precessing state the spin now has nonzero components perpendicular to the z axis (Fig. 2), or transverse to the main field. It is only the perpendicular (or transverse) components of the spin vector that give rise to a signal. Hence for image reconstruction it is only the projection of the 3D spin vector onto the 2D plane perpendicular to the z axis that

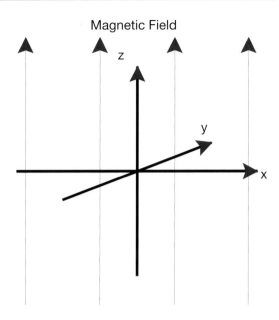

Fig. 1. Coordinate system aligned with the magnetic field

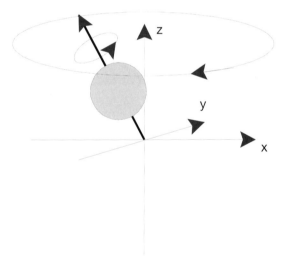

Fig. 2. A precessing spin

requires consideration. (Note, however, that when constructing imaging sequences, one must consider the full 3D nature of the spin, and its dynamics as described by the Bloch equations; see, for example, Slichter 1980.) The 2D projection of a 3D vector is illustrated in Figure 3.

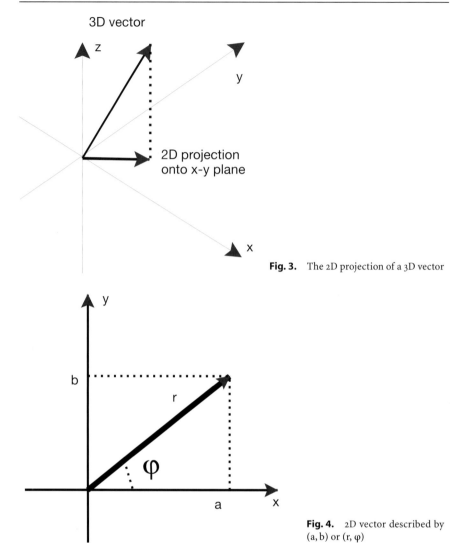

Fig. 3.   The 2D projection of a 3D vector

Fig. 4.   2D vector described by (a, b) or (r, φ)

2.2   Two-Dimensional Vectors and Complex Numbers

2D vectors can be described with respect to a cartesian coordinate system, as illustrated in Figure 4. A 2D vector requires two numbers to describe it. These can be either the vector's x and y components, or its length, and its angle with respect to the x axis. In terms of unit vectors in the x and y directions:

$$\left(\vec{\mathbf{x}}, \vec{\mathbf{y}} \right)$$

a general 2D vector can be expressed as:

$$\mathbf{v} = a\,\vec{\mathbf{x}} + b\,\vec{\mathbf{y}} \tag{1}$$

or using a=r cos(φ), and b=r sin(φ):

$$\mathbf{v} = r\,(\cos(\varphi)\,\vec{\mathbf{x}} + \sin(\varphi)\,\vec{\mathbf{y}}) \tag{2}$$

where a and b are the x and y components, respectively, and r and j are the length and angle, respectively. In MRI the projected spin vector is computed for each image element (pixel). For most imaging applications the orientation, φ (or phase), is not important. MR images typically display just the length (or magnitude) of the projection vector. (The most important exception to this is in phase contrast flow velocity imaging.)

While this vector concept is sufficient to fully describe MRI, the mathematics can become rather laborious. By utilizing a few notational tools a much more concise and powerful descriptive framework can be achieved. The first of these notational tools is complex numbers (see, for example, Morse and Feshbach 1953). Complex numbers are perfect for describing 2D vectors and their rotations in a plane. In fact complex numbers can be visualized graphically as 2D vectors. In analogy to x and y cartesian coordinates, a complex number can be described by a real and imaginary part, respectively, where i is used to distinguish the imaginary part from the real part. A complex number can be written as:

$$w = a + ib \tag{3}$$

or

$$w = r\big(\cos(\varphi) + i\sin(\varphi)\big) \tag{4}$$

The equations look similar to the vector Eqs. 1 and 2. Here, however, the x and y components depend implicitly on the absence or presence of i. Introducing the angular notation, exp($\iota\varphi$) = cos(φ) + isin(φ), Eq. 4 can be written:

$$w = r\exp\big(i\varphi\big) \tag{5}$$

which corresponds to the polar notation for complex numbers.

One important aspect about complex numbers is that ii = -1. As an example, the multiplication of two complex numbers proceeds as follows:

$$
\begin{aligned}
q &= w1.w2\\
&= (a + ib)(c + id)\\
&= ac + i(bc + ad) + iibd\\
&= (ac - bd) + i(bc + ad)
\end{aligned}
\tag{6}
$$

A further concept associated with complex numbers is that of the complex conjugate. The conjugate of a complex number is that number with the imaginary part negated. For instance the complex conjugate of w, in Eq. 3, is:

$$w^* = a - ib \tag{7}$$

where the asterisk indicates the complex conjugate of a complex number.

2.3 Complex Exponentials and Vector Rotation

Vector rotation requires a matrix multiplication. Expressing the vector in Eq. 1 as a column matrix, with the first and second elements corresponding to the x and y components, respectively, a rotation by an angle α can be calculated as follows:

$$\mathbf{q} = \begin{bmatrix} \cos(\alpha) & -\sin(\alpha) \\ \sin(\alpha) & \cos(\alpha) \end{bmatrix} \cdot \begin{bmatrix} a \\ b \end{bmatrix}$$
$$= \begin{bmatrix} a\cos(\alpha) - b\sin(\alpha) \\ a\sin(\alpha) + b\cos(\alpha) \end{bmatrix} \tag{8}$$

While this can rapidly become protracted with vectors, for complex numbers one simply multiples by $\exp(\iota\alpha)$. Starting with Eq. 5, and remembering that the product of exponentials is the same as the exponential of the sum of the exponents:

$$q = r\exp(i\varphi)\exp(i\alpha)$$
$$= r\exp(i(\varphi + \alpha)) \tag{9}$$

This can be confirmed starting with Eq. 4, and using some trigonometric identities:

$$q = r(\cos(\varphi) + i\sin(\varphi))(\cos(\alpha) + i\sin(\alpha))$$
$$= r((\cos(\varphi)\cos(\alpha) - \sin(\varphi)\sin(\alpha)) + i(\sin(\varphi)\cos(\alpha) + \cos(\varphi)\sin(\alpha)))$$
$$= r(\cos(\varphi + \alpha) + i\sin(\varphi + \alpha))$$
$$= r\exp(i(\varphi + \alpha)) \tag{10}$$

In truth this rotational example could have also been quite easily performed on the vector using the polar form. The real power of this technique becomes evident when the complex notation is coupled with Fourier transforms. Below it is seen how the spin rotations in the presence of a gradient field lead very naturally to the Fourier transform description of MRI.

2.4   Basics of 1D Fourier Transforms

The Fourier theory states that an object can be described equally well either by specifying its value directly at every point or indirectly by specifying it as the sum of a particular set of sine and cosine functions (see, for example, Bracewell 1978). Further, the Fourier theory describes how to calculate the particular set of sine and cosines for a given object. The sine and cosine description is generally known as the frequency domain (or frequency space) description; and the direct representation as the real domain (or real space) description. Fourier theory is well understood, and a frequency domain description can be converted to a real domain description (and visa versa) without loss of information.

A one-dimensional (1D) object can be described graphically as shown in Figure 5. The x axis represents the spatial (could also be time) coordinate, and the y axis displays the value of the particular object parameter under consideration. The curve indicates the parameter's value at a particular coordinate. The Fourier domain description can also be presented graphically. The curve in Figure 6 corresponds to that of Figure 5. This time, however, the x axis represents the frequency value of a component, and the y axis represents the strength (or weighting) of that frequency component. The object is constructed by summing all the frequency components represented by the graph. The curve here indicates with which weight each of the different frequency components should be applied to the sum constructing the object. Note that some frequency components are weighted negatively, which means that they are actually subtracted from the sum.

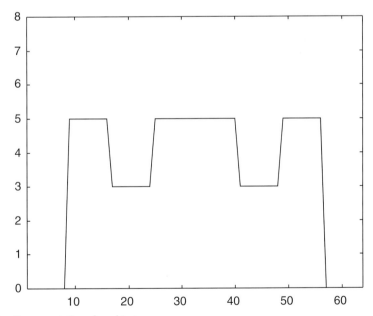

Fig. 5.   A "real" representation of an object

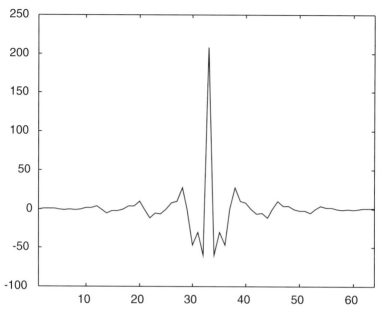

Fig. 6.   Frequency representation of the object in Figure 5

2.5   Fourier Construction of a 1D Box

To convey this idea of an object being composed of a number of frequency components, consider the construction of a boxlike object, shown in Figure 7. The first column represents a series of progressively accurate frequency domain descriptions. Each is composed, in this case, of discrete points. Each point represents a particular frequency. The points are displayed connected together. The second column shows the real domain approximate description of the object, which progressively improves as more and more frequency components are added to the frequency domain description. The third column show a series of real domain cosine waves and their weighting, corresponding to individual pairs of points in the frequency domain.

If the object is symmetrical, the y axis values describing the frequency weightings represent plain numbers. However, in the more general case the weighting factors are complex numbers. Here the magnitude of the complex value indicates the strength of the frequency component to be added. A nonzero phase value indicates that the frequency component needs to be shifted in the real domain before being summed. For a phase of 90° the shift is one-fourth of the wave period (which is called a shift of 90°), as shown in Figure 8. Thus complex numbers are also ideal for describing the weighting of the sinusoidal components of the Fourier transform.

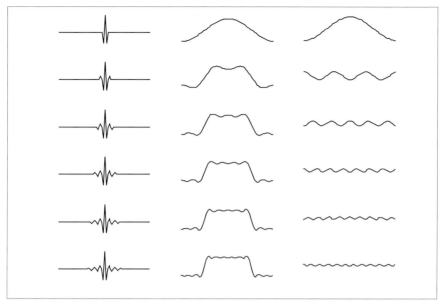

Fig. 7. The Fourier composition of a "box" object. *Left*, the Fourier description; *middle*, the object approximation; *right*, each additional individual frequency component

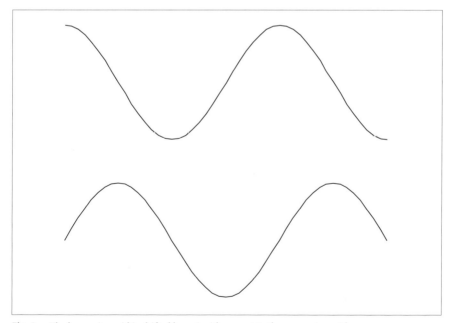

Fig. 8. The lower sinusoid is shifted by 90° with respect to the upper sinusoid

2.6   The Mathematics of Fourier Transforms

A Fourier transform is the operation of extracting the frequency domain description from the real domain description, and visa versa. Mathematically this is written as:

$$H(f) = \int_{-\infty}^{+\infty} h(x)\exp(-i2\pi\, fx)dx \tag{11}$$

where h(x) is the real domain object description, and H(f) is that for the frequency domain. H(f) and h(x) are both assumed to be complex valued. To understand this integral, consider that h(x), for a given position (x value), is a 2D vector. The term exp(–i2πfx) simply rotates this vector by an angle which, for a given frequency (f value), is proportional to x. The integral indicates that all the individually rotated vectors, for a given f value, are added up. Note that vectors pointing in different directions can cancel.

The term exp(–i2πfx) is known as an angular frequency. The minus sign is merely a convention and is not particularly significant for this discussion. As shown in Sect. 2.2, it is very closely related to the more familiar sine and cosine functions. A Fourier transform is a decomposition of an object into its angular frequency components. Assume h(x) can be represented by a single angular frequency (f_o), and a weighting (a). That is, h(x)=a exp(i2πf_ox). Then Eq. 11 becomes:

$$H(f) = a\int_{-\infty}^{+\infty} \exp(i2\pi\, f_o x)\exp(-i2\pi\, fx)\, dx$$

$$= a\int_{-\infty}^{+\infty} \exp(i2\pi(f_o - f)x)\, dx \tag{12}$$

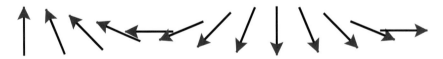

Fig. 9.   Vectors with linearly increasing rotational angle

The term in the integral now represents a unit length vector at every position x. However, the orientation angle (or phase angle) of the vector is a linear function of x, as shown in Figure 9. The rate of spatial variation is governed by (f_o–f). Now unless f_o=f, the orientation angles of all the vectors are equally distributed over 360°. Hence the vector sum tends to zero unless f_o=f (when all the vectors have the same orientation). Thus Eq. 12 becomes (neglecting the normalization constant from the infinite integral):

$$H(f) = a ; \quad f_o = f$$
$$= 0 ; \quad f_o \neq f \tag{13}$$

In other words, the Fourier transform determines the angular frequency component of our simple object h(x). This process also works when h(x) is composed of a very large number of frequency components (here the word angular is dropped from "angular frequency"; however, it is still implied).

There is also an inverse Fourier transform which recreates h(x) from H(f). This equation, very similar to Eq. 11 except for a minus sign and some reversing of roles, is:

$$h(x) = \int_{-\infty}^{+\infty} H(f) \exp(i2\pi fx) df \tag{14}$$

2.7   Aliasing or Undersampling

Frequently a discrete representation of an object is desired. If the representation is to be accurate, the sample spacing in the real domain must be structured suitably fine. Nyquist's theorem states that the sample spacing must be at least as fine as half the period of the highest frequency component within the object if the object representation is to be exact (see, for example, Bracewell 1978).

Theoretically for objects of finite extent this requirement means that all the frequency components from negative infinity to positive infinity are needed to describe the object with 100% accuracy. In practice, however, one must make do with less, by dealing with only a limited set of frequencies. In this case sampling is performed on a filtered representation of the object, where the filtering excludes the higher frequency components such that Nyquist's criterion is met.

There is also a sampling constraint in the frequency domain. It is actually identical to Nyquist's theorem. In this domain it translates into requiring that the sampling interval be equal to the reciprocal of the object's extent. Notice that because MRI deals with objects of finite extent, negative and positive infinities do not represent a problem in this domain.

In the event that the sampling interval in the frequency domain is not fine enough, the edges of the object are folded back onto the opposite edge of the object. This result of undersampling in the frequency domain is termed aliasing, and is illustrated in Figure 10. Figure 10 was created by starting with the top object, Fourier transforming it, removing every second sample point, and then inverse Fourier transforming the remaining data points. The resulting curve has the left half of the original added to the right side of the original, and the right half added to the left side.

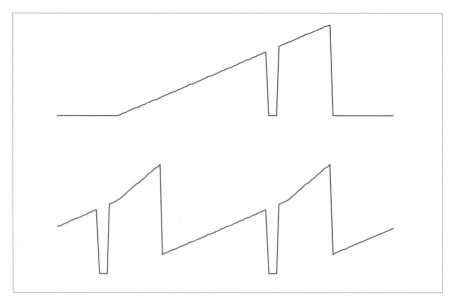

Fig. 10. The object at the top appears aliased (*bottom*) when its frequency space is sampled at less than the Nyquist rate

2.8   2D Fourier Transforms

Fourier transforms can be generalized for multidimensional objects. The only difficulty is that terms must be introduced to describe multidimensional frequencies. For spatial objects the term spatial frequency is used. The familiar temporal frequencies (describing time varying objects) are usually denoted by the variable f. However, for spatial frequencies (for objects in the spatial domain), k is generally used. For 2D spatial frequencies the coordinates k_x and k_y are introduced, corresponding to the x and y real object coordinates. The 2D Fourier transform contains a double integral because the integral is over an area, rather than along a line as in the case of the one dimensional object. The equation is:

$$H(k_x, k_y) = \int_{-\infty}^{+\infty}\int_{-\infty}^{+\infty} h(x, y)\exp(-i2\pi(xk_x + yk_y))dxdy \tag{15}$$

The extension for 3D objects follows (after introducing k_z) quite simply, and is given by:

$$H(k_x, k_y, k_z) = \int_{-\infty}^{+\infty}\int_{-\infty}^{+\infty}\int_{-\infty}^{+\infty} h(x, y, z)\exp(-i2\pi(xk_x + yk_y + zk_z))dxdydz \tag{16}$$

The inverse transforms are obtained in analogy to Eqs. 11 and 14.

2.9   2D Wave Functions

2D wave functions can be likened to waves on an ocean. In 1D frequency space the position represented the frequency of the wave. In 2D frequency space the position represents both the wave frequency and direction. Figure 11 displays the 2D wave function corresponding to several isolated points in the 2D frequency space. The further the point is located from the origin, the higher the frequency is. The orientation of the point with respect to the origin indicates the wave's direction.

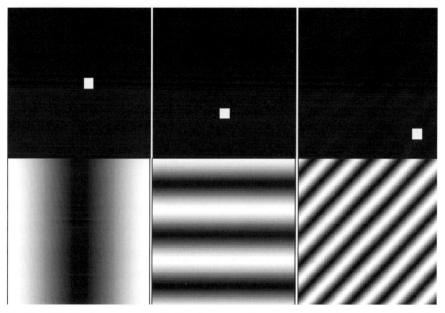

Fig. 11.   Points in frequency space (*top*) and corresponding representations in real space (*bottom*)

2.10   Fourier Construction of a 2D Object

The frequency representation of a bounded object extends to infinity in all directions. In MRI the frequency domain description of the object is measured. The problem is to create a good likeness of the object from data collected over only a limited region within the frequency domain. The appearance of an object reconstructed from several different bounded regions of frequency space is shown in Figure 12. Remember that the lower frequency terms are described near the origin of frequency space. The low frequency terms give a reasonable representation, but the fine details are missing. The higher frequency terms on their own, however, do not render a good image. The greater the extent, the better is the spatial resolution.

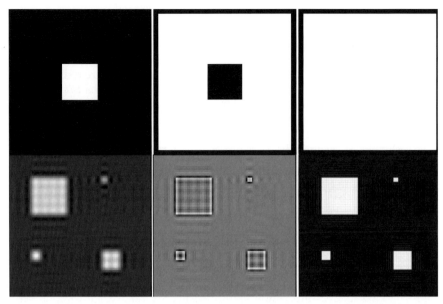

Fig. 12. Image appearance (*bottom*) depends on region of frequency space selected (*highlighted in white at top*)

In MRI the frequency space is measured over a region centered on the origin. The extent of the region depends on the desired spatial resolution. However, as becomes clearer below, measurement time increases with the area of the frequency space covered.

3   MRI Basics

This section considers MRI physics, commencing with resonance, moving on to gradient fields and pulse sequences, and ending with a mathematical description of the received signal.

3.1   Resonance

In nuclear magnetic resonance the spins precess (or rotate) about the z axis, which is aligned with the main magnetic field (B_0). The rotational frequency, f, is directly proportional to the field. That is:

$$f = \gamma \ B_0 \tag{17}$$

where γ is a proportionality constant, known as the gyromagnetic ratio. The key to MRI lies in varying the local magnetic field in a spatially dependent manner. In other words, the local resonance frequency is made to vary spatially.

3.2   Radiofrequency Field

Initially the spins are aligned along the z axis. In this state no MR signal is created. One purpose of the radiofrequency (RF) field is to rotate the spins into the x-y plane. An RF field has an oscillating (or rotating) magnetic field component, often denoted by B_1. To rotate the spins into the x-y plane B_1 needs to be perpendicular to the main field (B_0). This is achieved by the orientation of the RF coil. In addition to being perpendicular, B_1 must also oscillate (or rotate) at the precession frequency of the spins.

An RF pulse is a term indicating a short time period of a B_1 field activity. The strength of the B_1 field can be varied during the RF pulse to change the pulse's frequency characteristics. The most common requirement is to give the pulse a range of frequencies, rather than a single sharp resonance.

The angle through which the spins are rotated from the z axis towards the x-y plane depends on the strength of B_1 and the time over which it is applied. Thus the rotation angle depends on the total amount of RF energy applied. This is generally referred to as the flip angle of the RF pulse.

The RF field can be linearly or circularly polarized. This refers to an oscillating and rotating B_1 field, respectively. Spins interact with a field rotating in the same direction as their precession. However, as illustrated in Figure 13, a linearly polarized field can be considered as being composed of two counter rotating fields. In this case only one of the rotating fields interacts with the spins.

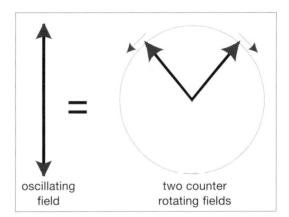

oscillating field = two counter rotating fields

Fig. 13.   Linear oscillation is identical to two counterrotating fields

3.3   Gradient Fields

Spatially dependent variations in the magnetic field are achieved with auxiliary magnet fields. These fields have their magnetic component aligned in the z direction (with the main magnetic field). However, the strength of the field varies spatially in a linear fashion. In addition, these auxiliary fields can be switched on and off. Thus the spatially dependent resonance frequency variations can be controlled dynamically. A gradient pulse is the term indicating a short time period

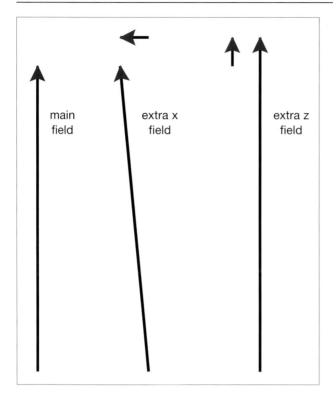

Fig. 14. Maximum change in length occurs if the auxiliary field is parallel to the main field

during which a gradient field is applied. As with an RF pulse, the strength can also be varied during the pulse.

The gradient field should be aligned with the main field, as this provides the maximum change in auxiliary field, and frequency, for a given gradient field. This is their purpose. The effect is illustrated in Figure 14. The total field is the vector sum of main and gradient field. Since the main field is about 500 times stronger than that caused by the gradient, there would be virtually no change in the magnitude of the total field if the magnetic component of the gradient field were perpendicular to that of the main field.

A schematic example of how a linear field gradient in the z direction can be achieved is shown in Figure 15. With counterrotating currents in the coils the field from one coil increases the magnetic field and the other decreases it. Between the two coils there is a more or less linear variation in field strength. Gradient coils for the x and y axes are slightly more complicated, as shown in Figure 16. On one side the field is increased, on the other it is reduced, and between them there is a more or less linear variation.

In the presence of gradient fields the local resonance frequency becomes:

$$f(x, y, z) = \gamma \left(B_0 + xG_x + yG_y + zG_z \right) \tag{18}$$

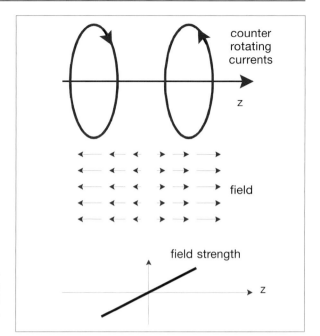

Fig. 15. Linear field gradient in z direction. *Top,* current carrying coils; *middle,* field between the coils; *bottom,* field strength verses z

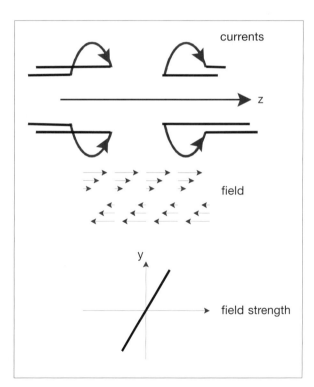

Fig. 16. Linear field gradient in y direction. *Top,* current carrying coils; *middle,* field between the coils; *bottom,* field strength verses y

where G_x, G_y, and G_z denote the gradient of the x, y, and z gradient fields, respectively. (When talking about gradient fields, their strength refers to the actual magnetic field gradient, not the magnetic field itself.) Notice, firstly, that the spatial dependencies are orthogonal, and, secondly, that they are linear. Other forms could have been chosen; however, this choice makes the imaging problem amenable to a Fourier transform solution.

3.4   Rotating Frame

When analyzing MRI experiments, it is the dynamically changing aspect of the resonance frequency which is important. The static portion determines the magnetization and hence the signal strength, but this is not important with respect to the spatial encoding for the image generation.

The rotating frame is a coordinate system, with its z axis aligned with that of stationary coordinate system. However, the rotating frame rotates about the z axis at a frequency given by γB_o ($= f_o$) (see Fig. 17). In this reference frame the precession frequency of the spins depends only on the gradient fields. That is:

$$f(x, y, z) = \gamma \left(xG_x + yG_y + zG_z \right) \tag{19}$$

In other words, in the absence of gradient fields, the spin is stationary. RF excitation is also easier to appreciate in the rotating frame, as the B_1 field no longer oscillates (or rotates).

A practical advantage of using Eq. 19, rather than 18, is that the frequencies are much reduced. This is more or less how MRI scanners operate. The measurement description takes place in the rotating frame. This is converted to the laboratory frame by increasing the RF pulse frequencies by f_o, and then the received data are converted back to the rotating frame by reducing their frequencies by f_o. This increasing and reducing is referred to as mixing or modulating.

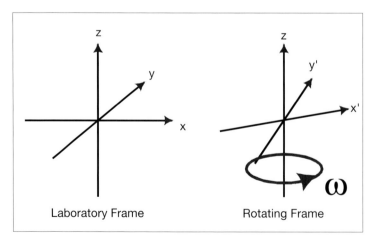

Fig. 17. The stationary and rotating coordinate frames

3.5   Spin Excitation in a Gradient Field

When a gradient field is applied, the resonance frequency within an object being imaged becomes a linear function of position (see Fig. 18). Assume that the spins are in their relaxed state, aligned with the z axis. If an RF pulse is applied, only those spins with a resonance frequency equal to the frequency of the RF pulse are rotated into the x-y plane. This rotation into the x-y plane is known as excitation. (MR signal is generated only by excited spins.) Thus the act of applying an RF pulse in the presence of a gradient field is to excite a set of spins lying in a plane corresponding to a particular resonance frequency. This is the basis of slice selection. For instance, referring to Figure 18, if the frequency of the RF pulse is 20 kHz (in the rotating frame), only the spins with a 20 kHz resonance frequency (in the rotating frame) are excited.

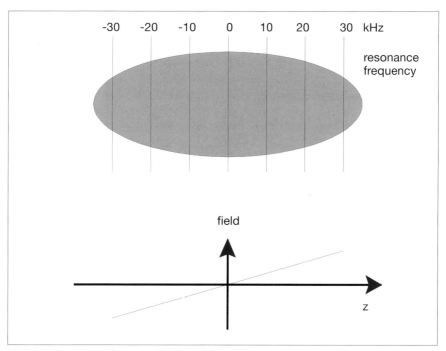

Fig. 18.   The resonant frequency distribution during slice selection

3.6   Signal Detection in a Gradient Field

Assume that a set of spins has been excited and is precessing in the x-y plane. If a field gradient is applied, the precession frequency becomes a function of position (see Fig. 19). If the signal is sampled and a frequency analysis performed, a

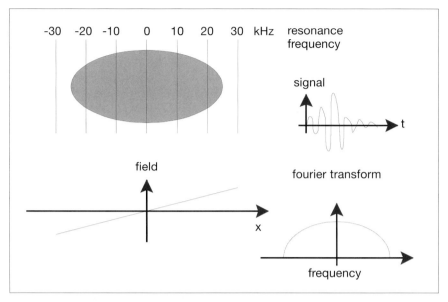

Fig. 19. Signal detection with a gradient field

particular frequency component of the signal can be assigned to have originated from a plane within the object corresponding to the particular resonance frequency. If the excitation and detection gradient fields are orthogonal, the particular frequency components can be assigned as to having originated from the line of intersection of the two planes. This is called frequency encoding and is one of the steps required for producing an MR image.

3.7   Spin Precession in a Gradient Field

The third situation to be considered is that in which a gradient field is switched on and then off again after a predetermined length of time. Assume that the spins have been excited and are now precessing in the x-y plane. Initially in the absence of gradient fields (and in the rotating frame) they are all stationary and in phase. If a gradient field is applied, the resonance frequency becomes spatially dependent, and the spins start to precess at different rates (see Fig. 20). If the gradient field is removed, each spin will have acquired a phase which depends on the resonance frequency, in the presence of the gradient field, multiplied by the length of time that the gradient field was applied. Since the gradient field renders the resonance frequency spatially dependent, the phase acquired by the spins is also a function of position. Thus the phase of the signal allows it to be assigned to a particular plane within the object. For a single measurement this assignment is ambiguous. A series of measurements with different gradient field strengths is required to overcome this, as is explained below.

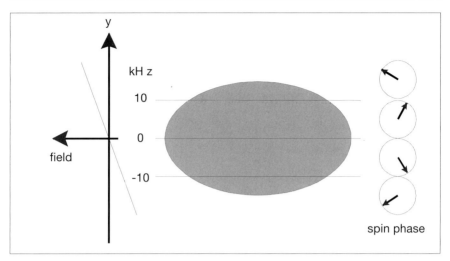

Fig. 20. Spin phase accumulation due to a gradient pulse

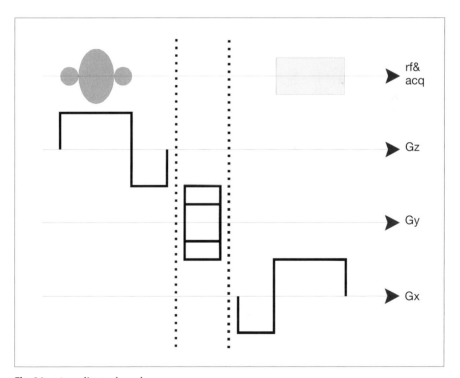

Fig. 21. A gradient-echo pulse sequence

3.8   A Pulse Sequence Diagram

A pulse sequence diagram is a powerful graphic tool for describing an MRI experiment. An example of a gradient-echo sequence is shown in Figure 21. Time proceeds from left to right. The top curve indicates both the time course of the RF field and the period of time during which the MR signal is acquired. The next three curves indicate the gradient produced by the respective gradient fields as a function of time. Note that points aligned vertically occur at the same point in time. Figure 21 has been divided into three segments. These represent the three steps towards acquiring data suitable for converting into an MR image. The next few sections focus on these steps in more detail.

In actual fact a waiting period is added after the acquisition period, since time is generally allotted for the spins to realign themselves towards the z axis, prior to the next excitation. However, for the present goal of deriving the imaging equations, this waiting period can safely be ignored. For fast MRI the sequence should be shortened as much as possible. As the influence of gradient fields on the spin phase is linear, gradient pulses between the RF pulse and acquisition period can be overlapped, as shown in Figure 22. There are many different pulse sequences in MRI. That shown is Figure 22 is probably the simplest.

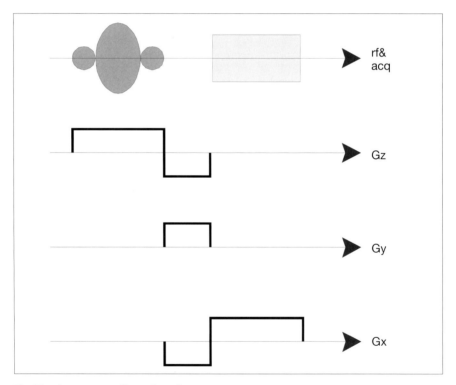

Fig. 22.   A compact gradient-echo pulse sequence

3.9   Slice Selection

The slice selection segment is shown in Figure 23. The characteristics of the RF pulse include a center frequency, f_{rf}, and a bandwidth, bw_{rf}. The RF pulse is composed of a range of frequencies. The strength of each of the frequency components within the range is usually more or less equal. The range of frequencies is centered on f_{rf}, and their extent is indicated by bw_{rf}. The slice selection gradient (the positive gradient pulse) has an amplitude (or strength), G_s, and is followed by a rephasing gradient pulse, with opposite sign. Immediately following the RF pulse the spins within the slice have a phase which varies linearly through the slice. The purpose of the rephasing gradient is to realign the spins so that they all have the same phase. This leads to maximum signal.

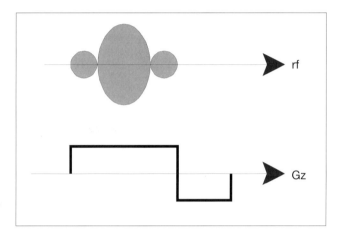

Fig. 23.   The slice selection segment

Often one speaks about a gradient area. This refers to the product of gradient strength and the length of time during which the gradient is active. The area is a measure for the amount of phase variation caused by the gradient per unit length. The area of the rephasing gradient should be approximately equal to the product of G_s and the time interval from the center of the RF pulse to the end of the slice selection gradient. The position of the selected slice is given by:

$$z_s = f_{rf} / \gamma \, G_s \qquad\qquad (20)$$

and the thickness of the selected slice is given by:

$$\Delta z = bw_{rf} / \gamma \, G_s \qquad\qquad (21)$$

Typically, for fast imaging at least, bw_{rf} is set as high as possible (compatible with patient safety and hardware constraints), G_s is determined from Eq. 21 using the desired slice thickness, and finally f_s is calculated depending on Eq. 20 and the desired slice position.

3.10 Phase Encoding

The purpose of the phase-encoding gradient pulse is to impart a spatially dependent phase to the spins. The pulse is sometimes drawn to indicate that the amplitude is varied from measurement to measurement (Fig. 24). If the maximum strength is denoted G_p, and a spatial resolution δ is required, the length of the pulse is:

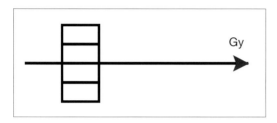

Fig. 24. The (variable amplitude) phase-encoding gradient

$$T_p = 1 / \gamma\, G_p \delta \tag{22}$$

The pulse amplitude is varied from $-G_p$ to $+G_p$, in N steps; where N is the dimension of the image matrix. The field of view (FOV) then is given as:

$$FOV = N\delta \tag{23}$$

Defining the parameter n as varying from $-(N-1)/2$ to $N/2$, and denoting the gradient amplitude step by g_p $(= 2G_p/N)$, the phase shift for the n'th measurement is given by:

$$\varphi = \gamma\, nT_p g_p\, y \tag{24}$$

where this gradient is assumed to be in the y direction.

3.11 Frequency Encoding

The final element in the imaging sequence is the frequency encoding (see Fig. 25). There is a period T_f over which data are acquired. During this period the frequency-encoding gradient of strength G_f is applied. Prior to the frequency-encoding gradient the prephasing gradient is positioned. This imparts a spatially dependent phase variation to the spins, which is subsequently undone by the frequency-encoding gradient. The area of the prephasing gradient amounts to exactly half the area of the frequency-encoding gradient. This ensures that the spins are then all realigned (or in phase) at the center of the acquisition period. The sampling rate, f_s, during signal acquisition is:

$$f_s = \gamma\, G_f\, FOV \tag{25}$$

and the acquisition period is:

$$T_f = 1 / \gamma\, G_f \delta \tag{26}$$

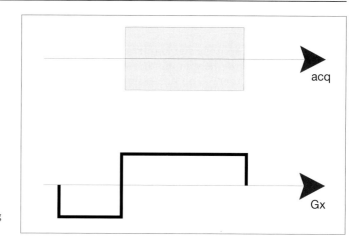

Fig. 25. The
frequency-encoding
segment

where δ is, again, the spatial resolution. The purpose here is to produce a spatially dependent precession frequency which, using Eq. 19, is given by:

$$f = \gamma \, G_f x \qquad (27)$$

3.12 Signal Reception

The 2D transverse spin vector acts as a small bar magnet. For a 1-T scanner this vector precesses at about 42 MHz. As with an electric generator, the precessing spin induces an electric current in conducting coils placed nearby. This current, which is subsequently amplified in the receiver, constitutes the MR signal.

MRI coils are not focused in any way. Hence they detect all signals in their vicinity. The sensitivity of these coils decreases as the distance between the coil and spin increases however.

The signal in the MR receiver is a real signal. It thus does not require complex numbers to describe it. It is merely a current going back and forth. As discussed in Sect. 3.2, a real signal, being basically a linear oscillation, can be considered as a sum of two counterrotating components. Only one corresponds to the direction of the spin precession. This rotating component can be extracted from the real signal, either electronically or numerically. As a consequence complex numbers are now required to describe the resultant signal.

When the generation is performed electronically, two real signals are generated. However, one corresponds to the real part and the other to the imaginary part. These are known as in-phase and quadrature signals, respectively. After sampling, the two signals are combined to produce a numerical complex signal description. The important point here is that the complex signal description has a direct relationship to the complex spin description.

3.13   The MRI Signal

For a single excited spin the signal mirrors (or is equivalent to) the complex description of the state of the spin vector over time. In the rotating frame, and without gradient fields, there is no precession. Thus, ignoring all sorts of scale factors, the signal is identical to the transverse spin vector. That is:

$$s(t) = \rho \tag{28}$$

where ρ represents the length of the spin vector. The spin vector is assumed to be orientated along the x axis (that is it has a phase angle of zero); and relaxation effects are ignored.

Suppose now that a phase-encoding gradient was applied prior to the period in which the signal is being observed. Making use of complex exponentials to denote 2D vector rotation, the spin acquires a phase given by Eq. 24. Thus for the n`th measurement:

$$s_n(t) = \rho(y_0) \exp(i2\pi\gamma\, nT_p g_p y_0) \tag{29}$$

for a spin located at y_0. For the moment the spin is still stationary. This changes when the frequency-encoding gradient is added. Now the spin phase changes with time. Noting that the phase is equal to the product of precession frequency (Eq. 27) and time, the signal becomes:

$$s_n(t) = \rho(x_0, y_0) \exp(i2\pi\gamma\, nT_p g_p y_0) \exp(i2\pi\gamma\, G_x x_0 t)$$
$$= \rho(x_0, y_0) \exp(i2\pi\gamma\,(nT_p g_p y_0 + G_x x_0 t)) \tag{30}$$

where the origin of the time variable, t, is defined as being that point in the center of the acquisition period where the spins all have the same phase. Now both the x and y coordinates of the spin are required.

The total received signal corresponds to the sum of all signals from the individual spins. Mathematically this is described by a 2D integral over x and y. Hence the received signal can be described by the equation:

$$s_n(t) = \int_{-\infty}^{+\infty}\int_{-\infty}^{+\infty} \rho(x, y) \exp(i2\pi\gamma\,(nT_p g_p y + G_x xt))\, dx\, dy \tag{31}$$

The imaging problem is to recover the 2D spin distribution $\rho(x, y)$ from the set of measured signals $s_n(t)$.

4   k-Space

k-space is a very powerful concept in MRI, as it provides a solid framework both for designing MRI experiments and for understanding imaging artifacts (Twieg 1983; Ljunggren 1983). In the early stages of MRI this framework was not available, and knowing the most suitable set of experiments to perform, as well as how to reconstruct an image from a given set of data, was poorly understood.

k-Space is based on a Fourier description of the MRI process.

4.1 Equations

k-Space follows in a straightforward fashion from Eq. 31. The idea is to turn this into a 2D Fourier transform. Firstly define two new variables:

$$k_x = \gamma \, G_x t \tag{32}$$

and:

$$k_y = \gamma \, ng_p T_p \tag{33}$$

Also note that $s_n(t)$ is a function of the two parameters, t and n, which are scaled version of k_x and k_y. Thus by suitably stretching and/or compressing the coordinates of $s_n(t)$, the 2D function $S(k_x,k_y)$ can be obtained. Using Eqs. 32 and 33, this becomes:

$$S(k_x, k_y) = \int_{-\infty}^{+\infty}\int_{-\infty}^{+\infty} \rho(x, y) \exp(i2\pi \, (k_x x + k_y y)) \, dx \, dy \tag{34}$$

which is equivalent to the inverse 2D Fourier transform corresponding to Eq. 15. The image of the spin distribution is obtained by the Fourier transform:

$$\rho(x, y) = \int_{-\infty}^{+\infty}\int_{-\infty}^{+\infty} S(k_x, k_y) \exp(-i2\pi \, (k_x x + k_y y)) \, dk_x \, dk_y \tag{35}$$

Thus k-space is none other than the spatial frequency domain. Another key towards understanding MRI is appreciating that the object being imaged is sampled in the spatial frequency domain. Thus the frequency domain sampling requirements, discussed in Sect. 2.7, apply here as well.

Note that k-space is acquired line by line. A line of k_x points, for a given k_y value, is acquired with each individual measurement.

4.2 Image Signal to Noise Ratio

k-Space can also be used to understand signal to noise influences on the image. The signal is directly proportional to the volume of the image element. Denoting the x and y pixel dimensions by δ_x and δ_y, respectively (slice thickness is Δz), the signal in a pixel is proportional to $\delta_x \delta_y \Delta z$.

Assume that there are N_x and N_y samples in the k_x and k_y directions, respectively. The full signal bandwidth (bw_s) determines the sampling rate (f_s), which is set according to the Nyquist criterion. Note that the frequencies present extend from $-f_s/2$ to $+f_s/2$, and that the maximum frequency is thus $f_s/2$. For this reason $f_s/2$ is sometimes used for the signal (and sampling) bandwidth. Here, however, f_s is used.

The noise per unit bandwidth is a constant (depending on patient and coil). It is assumed to be a random process. The expected (in a statistical sense) value for the magnitude of a sum of noise values is equal to the square root of the number of samples multiplied by the expected value of the noise for a single sample. Thus the noise per k-space point is proportional to $\sqrt{bw_s}$. Knowing how k-space noise contributes to image noise is equivalent to determining what a Fourier transform does to a random signal. Note that if the sampling rate exceeds the full signal bandwidth, noise is not completely random between k-space samples.

If a signal is random, from a statistical view point, the phase of the exponential term within the Fourier transform is irrelevant. Statistically, with respect to the noise the Fourier transform acts as a simple summation. Thus if the expectation value of the noise per sample is n, the expectation value of the Fourier transform of N noise samples is $n\sqrt{N}$.

The signal values on Fourier transforming add up directly and thus increase by N. Hence the signal to noise ratio after the Fourier transform in the k_x direction is:

$$SNR_{1D} \propto \frac{\delta_x \delta_y \Delta z\, N_x}{\sqrt{bw_s N_x}}$$

$$= \frac{\delta_x \delta_y \Delta z}{\sqrt{\left(bw_s / N_x\right)}} \tag{36}$$

The term bw_s/N_x represents the bandwidth per pixel. Denote this by bw_p. For a 2D Fourier transform this process is repeated in the second coordinate direction. Hence the signal to noise ratio in an image is:

$$SNR_{2D} \propto \frac{\delta_x \delta_y \Delta z\, N_y}{\sqrt{bw_p N_y}}$$

$$= \frac{\delta_x \delta_y \Delta z\, \sqrt{N_y}}{\sqrt{bw_p}} \tag{37}$$

5   k-Space Considerations for Ultrafast Imaging

5.1   k-Space Coverage and Image Resolution

The larger the extent of the k-space coverage, the higher is the image resolution. The extent of k-space is controlled (see Eqs. 32, 33) by the areas of the phase-encoding and frequency-encoding gradients. Hence higher resolution imaging sequences require more time.

5.2   K-Space Coverage and Field of View

The Nyquist requirement (Sect. 2.7) dictates the sample spacing in k-space. For spatial resolution to remain the same, an increase in the field of view requires the data to be acquired on a finer grid. The extent of the k-space coverage remains the same.

There is no time or signal to noise penalty in sampling k_x at a higher rate (that is on a finer grid). There is only more data to process. However, sampling k_y on a finer grid requires additional phase-encoding measurements, and this increases the total imaging time. In other words, increasing the field of view coverage in the phase-encoding direction for the same spatial resolution increases the measurement time. Note that the extra measurements improve the signal to noise according to Eq. 37.

Undersampling in the k_y direction in an attempt to reduce imaging time is the primary cause of image aliasing in MRI. This happens when the size of the field of view in the phase-encoding direction is too small.

5.3   Fractional K-Space Imaging

It turns out that if the spin phase is everywhere zero, the k-space representation of the image has the property that one half of k-space is the complex conjugate (see Eq. 7) of the other. More exactly:

$$S(k_x, k_y) = S^*(-k_x, -k_y) \tag{38}$$

The implication of this is that if half of the k-space representation is known, the other half can be generated numerically, without any loss in image resolution. The spin phase being everywhere a constant could also be tolerated, as a constant phase could easily be removed.

Due to main magnetic field inhomogeneities and eddy current induced fields, in practice the spin phase is not everywhere the same. In many situations, however, the spatial variation of the phase is slight and hence can be estimated with a low-resolution image. Typically approx. 55% of k-space is acquired, and the central 10% used to determine the low-frequency phase variation. This is used to correct the measured data before estimating the missing components.

For ultrafast imaging fractional k-space acquisitions should be used. The exceptions are gradient-echo imaging with long echo times and phase-contrast MRI. Field inhomogeneities and velocity encoding, respectively, produce significant spatially dependent phase variations such that Eq. 38 no longer applies (even approximately).

The penalty of half k-space imaging is a reduction in the signal to noise ratio. However the imaging time can be almost halved. Another minor issue is that reconstruction of fractional k-space acquired data takes slightly longer.

5.4   Half-Echo Verses Half-Nex

There are two ways of acquiring fractional k-space data. Generally each line of k-space is acquired symmetrically about the k_y axis. Each line of data is known as an echo. With half-echo imaging only the left or right half of k-space is measured, by acquiring only about 55% of the k_x samples. This reduces the time required for each measurement. A second advantage of half-echo acquisitions is that the echo time is reduced, which has a very beneficial effect with respect to imaging vessels containing turbulent flow. With very short echo times the chance of turbulence induced signal voids is reduced. Moving spins undergo a velocity-dependent phase shift. With turbulence the spin velocities can be very different, hence the phase dispersal can be large. Fortunately, however, the phase shift depends on the echo time.

The other approach to acquiring fractional k-space data involves collecting only those k-space lines in the top or bottom half of k-space. This means that only about 55% of the acquisitions are required. The strategy is generally referred to as a half k-space, or half-nex, acquisition. ("nex" is an abbreviation for number of excitations.)

In ultrafast imaging the sampling bandwidth is relatively high in order to reduce the sequence time. Hence the data acquisition (readout) period is not much longer than the time required to apply the RF excitation pulse and slice selection gradient. In this regime halving the number of excitations results in a much greater reduction in total image acquisition time compared with collecting just half-echos.

Note that combining both half-echo and half-nex in one acquisition results in resolution loss.

5.5   View Sharing

This is a technique which can be employed to enhance temporal resolution. Typically, temporal changes in the depicted object are due to the passage of contrast, cardiac or respiratory motion, or the act of moving the imaging plane during scanning.

For these types of dynamic imaging situations, k-space data is repeatedly acquired. Conventionally an image reconstruction is started each time a new set of k-space data is present. Thus the imaging rate equals the k-space acquisition rate. With view sharing, however, image reconstruction is started several times during a k-space acquisition cycle, as illustrated in Figure 26. Hence each image is reconstructed using k-space views which are shared with other images. While this increases the imaging rate, it does not increase temporal resolution. The temporal resolution is determined by the time required to obtain a full set of k-space data. In effect one ends up with an interpolated set of images which smooth the transitions from one point to another.

There are many strategies regarding the order in which k-space data should be collected. For smooth transitions between view shared images, the k-space data should be acquired in an interleaved (or interlaced) manner (see Fig. 27),

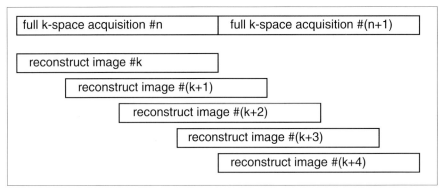

Fig. 26. With view sharing, images are reconstructed more often than a full set of k-space data is collected

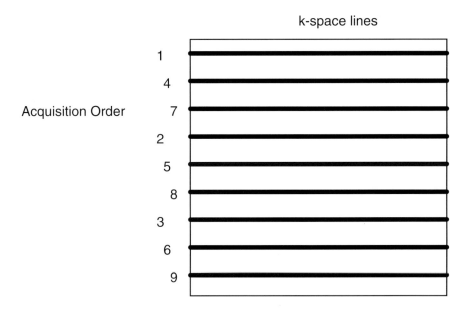

Fig. 27. For view sharing the k-lines are acquired in an interleaved manner

with the imaging rate synchronized with the time to acquire one or multiple interleaves of k-space data. However for monitoring lower resolution changes more rapidly, often the central k-space lines (those corresponding to the low resolution image content) are collected more often than the outer k-space lines.

View sharing has the potential for significantly improving the imaging of contrast kinetics.

5.6   Zero Filling

Zero filling is a data processing step (Du et al. 1994). Hence it requires no additional data collection time. Zero filling appears to increase the image resolution; however, it is really just a better interpolation technique. MR images are typically acquired with an acquisition matrix of 256 × 256 or slightly less, and reconstructed to an image matrix of 256 × 256. This is not the best way to display data acquired from structures with dimensions in the order of a pixel of less. (In practice the image may be linearly interpolated to a 512 × 512 matrix. However this does not change the following argument.)

In a simplified sense the amplitude of an image pixel is the sum of the signal from within a voxel. This would indicate that a very small signal source within a voxel would appear the same irrespective of its location within the voxel. However, this is not strictly the case.

The amplitude of a pixel is equal to the convolution of signal producing objects with a peaked function with roughly the dimensions of a pixel, sampled at points on a grid. (The peaked function would be, for instance, a sinc function in the absence of k-space windowing.) Now in this scenario the appearance of a small object depends on the position of the object with respect to the sampling grid.

In the above scenario the sampling grid (the image matrix) is of the same order as the acquisition matrix. Zero filling is nothing more than calculating the image on a finer sampling grid. Mathematically it is a form of interpolation tai-

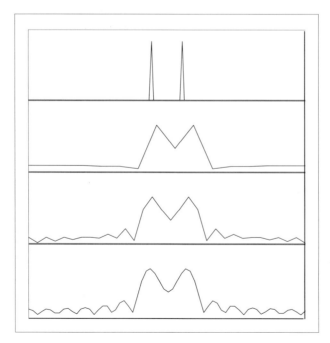

Fig. 28. Two closely spaced points (*top*), and their appearance with no zero filling, a zero filling factor of 2, and 4 (*bottom*) respectively

lored to the Fourier reconstruction. Practically it is achieved by extending the data matrix with zeros, requiring an increase in the size of the Fourier transform, which in turn produces a finer image grid. Typically the sample points are doubled in each image dimension. An example of this effect is shown in Figure 28. Two pointlike objects are sampled at slightly more than the Nyquist rate, and then displayed without zero filling and after doubling and quadrupling the data matrix via zero filling. Note that with zero filling the two objects are better resolved, and their displayed position is more accurate.

Angiographic images exhibit a marked improvement with zero filling. The reason is that the maximum intensity projection is typically calculated using the noninterpolated image matrix. For 3D data sets the amount of data to be reconstructed is increased by a factor of eight with zero filling, which increases data storage requirements and processing times considerably.

The apparent resolution increase means that the actual acquisition matrix can be reduced, which in turn has a considerable impact on 3D imaging times.

6   Coherence Pathways

A key aspect of designing fast imaging sequences is an appreciation of coherence pathways (Hennig 1988). Magnetization, after it has been excited by an RF pulse, evolves. Spins precess at a rate determined by the local magnetic field. Now, ignoring relaxation for the moment, every time an RF pulse is applied, excited magnetization does one of just five things:
a) A part continues to precess as though nothing had happened.
b) A part is placed into the z direction where it stops precessing.
c) A part is refocused (or in other words its phase is conjugated). These first three processes apply to excited magnetization lying in the x-y plane prior to an RF pulse. For excited magnetization aligned along the z axis prior to an RF pulse:
d) a part can remain aligned with the z axis, and
e) another part can be brought into the x-y plane, and hence continue to precess.

The distribution of magnetization into the different components is controlled largely by the flip angle of the RF pulses.

Thus every time an RF pulse is applied the magnetization is split into differently evolving fractions. Each of these differently evolving fractions is called a coherence pathway. Coherence, in the sense used here, can be thought of as the particular phase evolution of a given set of spins.

In situations where the T2 relaxation is short compared to the time between RF pulses, only the initial magnetization need be considered. However, with rapid imaging sequences this is seldom the case. Generally magnetization that is excited by several different prior RF pulses is present in each acquired signal. In the early days of rapid imaging this caused interesting image artifacts. However, this is now well understood.

6.1 Controlling the Coherences

The problem associated with the presence of many different coherence pathway signals (or coherences) in the acquired signal, is that each coherence potentially has a different phase. Thus there can be strong interference effects, with signal enhancement or cancellation in different regions of the image.

One remedy is to dephase the unwanted coherences. This involves applying a sufficiently large gradient pulse after the signal acquisition such that the spin phase within a voxel is distributed over 720° or greater. To avoid eventually refocusing certain coherences the amount of dephasing must be varied from acquisition to acquisition. It is difficult to keep track of the different coherence pathways or to determine the optimum sequence of dephasing gradient pulses to be used. Also, the length of the dephasing gradient pulse is proportional to the number of coherence pathways to be suppressed, and these increase exponentially with the number of RF pulses.

The only means to control the coherences is to make sure that the spin evolution during any pair of RF pulses (for spins in the x-y plane) is a constant depending only on spatial position. This is the reason why gradient-recalled echo sequences require a rewinder gradient pulse to counter the effect of the phase-encoding pulse.

A second step towards controlling the coherences lies in assuring that the spin evolution be sufficiently large such that the signal is dephased after each acquisition. This second requirement means that only the initial and the refocused coherences contribute to the acquired signal. The first requirement also means that the RF pulse spacing be constant.

Note that the spin evolution is different at different spatial locations due to the inhomogeneities in the main magnetic field. The second requirement eliminates possible interference artifacts due to field inhomogeneities. With extremely short repetition times this requirement could be relaxed.

6.2 Coherence Pathway Diagram

Given the two requirements of constant and sufficient evolution per RF pulse interval, the coherence pathways can be illustrated as shown in Figure 29. Spin phase is plotted verses time for all the coherence pathways at a given spatial position. At every RF pulse the coherence pathways are further split. Refocusing, or conjugating, the magnetization is equivalent to negating the spin phase. Note that the solid lines indicate spins in the x-y plane, while the dotted lines display those in the z direction. This diagram only depicts the coherence pathway for magnetization excited by the first RF pulse. For a complete picture this pattern needs to be repeated for each RF pulse. The magnetization contributing to the signal is that crossing the zero phase axis. The magnetization away from this axis is assumed to be dephased. The main point of Figure 29 is to show the large number of potential coherence pathways present. However, it can also be used when numerically calculating the image contrast and signal levels once the equations for the pathway splitting and the relaxation are incorporated.

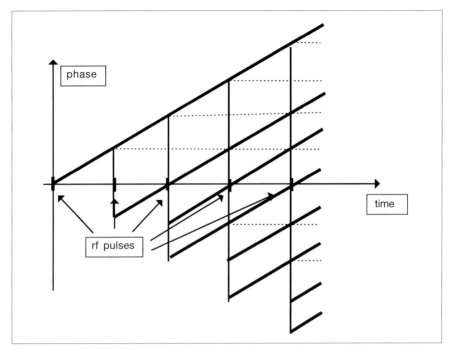

Fig. 29. The coherence build up and evolution for equally spaced RF pulses

7   Fast Gradient-Echo Imaging

The basic gradient-echo imaging sequence was discussed in Sect. 3 (Fig. 22; see, for example, van der Meulen 1988). The key to dealing with the multiple coherence pathways is to add a rewinder gradient for constant evolution and to extend the readout gradient for sufficient dephasing. This is shown in Figure 30. The area of the rewinder is equal to that of the phase-encoding gradient, but it has the opposite polarity.

7.1   Refocused Gradient-Echo Imaging

Figure 30 could perhaps best be denoted as a refocused gradient-echo imaging sequence. However, depending on the manufacturer, it is referred to as FLASH, FFE, or GRASS. This sequence has a complex contrast behavior. For short repetition times the contrast is primarily T_1 dependent. Regions with a short T_1 appear bright. However, in regions where T_2 is long the different coherences persist longer, and thus there is also a T_2-weighted signal enhancement.

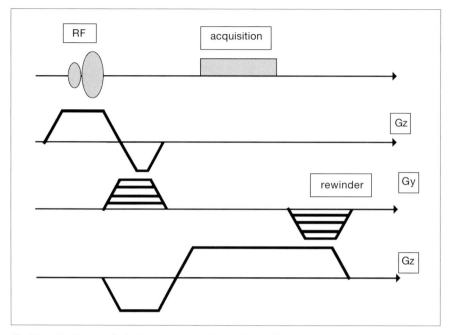

Fig. 30. Gradient-recalled echo sequence with rewinder gradient

Even with very short repetition times multiple refocusing of coherences provides a reasonable signal to noise ratio for refocused gradient-echo sequences. Its poor contrast characteristics limit its use however.

7.2 Spoiled Gradient-Echo Imaging

In order to obtain a pure T1, weighting the signal from all coherences, other than the primary excited magnetization following the RF pulse, needs to be destroyed (or spoiled). Initially this was tried by pseudo-randomly varying the phase evolution between two RF pulses either by using dephasing gradient pulses of varying area or by varying the phase of the RF pulse itself. Changing the phase of the RF pulse implies that the direction of the B1 field in the x-y plane (of the rotating frame) is changed. Thus the phase of the excited signal is also changed. This phase shift must be removed from the acquired signal before or during the image reconstruction processing. However, as phase can be controlled, this is a well-known value. It can be removed either electronically by changing the receiver phase or numerically on the digital data. The random phase addition to the coherences causes them to destructively interfere. However, there is still significant signal left, and this appears as a low-level additional background noise spread over the image in the phase-encoding direction.

Today a coherent type of spoiling is usually employed. The goal is to choose the RF phase shifts such that the multiple coherence pathway signals actually cancel each other. To do this in a controlled manner it is necessary that the phase evolution between any pair of RF pulses be controlled (Zur et al. 1991). For phase spoiling the phase angle difference between two neighboring RF pulses should increase linearly with pulse number. Using numerical simulations it has been found that values such as 117° and 123°, for the rate of increase, work very well.

7.3   Reaching Steady State

Making an image requires that multiple lines of k-space data be acquired. However, the signal collected by the initial acquisitions is very different from that collected by later acquisitions. There are two reasons for this. Firstly, the coherence pathways require several RF pulses before they are established. Thus the first acquisition consists of only one coherence, the second also has only one, the third has two, and the fourth and fifth have three and five, respectively. Thereafter it rapidly becomes more complicated. Eventually each acquisition collects a fairly similar set of coherences. This situation is denoted as the coherence steady state.

The second aspect is the initial excited magnetization. For the first RF pulse the full thermal equilibrium magnetization is available. However, for the second the magnetization available is simply the sum of that remaining following the first pulse plus the magnetization that has recovered due to T_1 relaxation between RF pulses. The third RF pulse contains even less signal to start with. Eventually the unexcited z magnetization is reduced to a point at which the component converted into excited (x, y) magnetization equals that which recovers between RF pulses. At this point the longitudinal magnetization steady state is reached.

In a pure sense, a steady state for both the coherence and longitudinal magnetization is never truly reached. However eventually the signal variation from acquisition to acquisition becomes negligible, at least with respect to image artifacts. Typically this pragmatic definition is what is implied by steady state.

Most imaging sequences use a number of prior preparatory acquisitions, which are identical to the imaging acquisitions except that no data are collected. The preparatory acquisitions are used to drive the spin system closer towards the steady state before acquiring the signals to be used in the image reconstruction. This is to prevent or reduce artifacts due to varying magnetization levels. As the magnetization variations have more effect on the image appearance if they occur during the central k-space acquisitions, typically the acquisitions are started at the edge of k-space rather than in the center. Thus the magnetization has a chance to settle down before the central k-space data lines are collected.

7.4   Designing a Fast Gradient-Recalled Echo Sequence

In this section the equations involved in determining the minimum sequence time for gradient-recalled echo imaging are discussed.

7.4.1   Gradients

Let G_m and G_s denote the maximum gradient amplitude and slew rate, respectively. Slew rate denotes the speed at which the gradient strength can be changed. The rise time (RT), or time required to switch the gradients from off to full on, is given by:

$$RT=G_m/G_s \tag{39}$$

7.4.2   RF Pulse

For low flip angle imaging a sinc type pulse can be assumed. The period of the sinc function (T_s) is determined by the pulse bandwidth (bw_{rf}):

$$T_s=2/bw_{rf} \tag{40}$$

However the total length of the pulse depends on the number of sinc periods uses. The more periods are incorporated, the better is the slice definition. Typically for rapid imaging, however, only the central lobe and one prelobe (or 1.5 periods) are used, as shown in Figure 30. This is sometimes known as a truncated sinc pulse. Using Eq. 21:

$$bw_{rf} = \Delta z \gamma\, G_m \tag{41}$$

In this case RF power deposition in the patient must be watched. A high RF bandwidth implies a high peak RF energy. However, for reduced flip angle imaging the RF bandwidth can be made higher than normal, as the energy for a given pulse scales as the square of the flip angle.

The effect of the slice-selective rephasing gradient lobe on the overall repetition time can usually be ignored when a truncated sinc pulse is used. Also, the phase-encoding gradient is typically shorter than the readout prephasing gradient lobe and can likewise be ignored for this analysis.

7.4.3   Acquisition

The length of the acquisition period (T_a) is (from Eq. 26):

$$T_a = 1/\gamma\, G_m \delta\, x \tag{42}$$

This is for a full-echo acquisition. When coupled with a half-nex fractional k-space acquisition the shortest imaging time results. The time for the readout prephaser requires half the area of the acquisition gradient. Also the readout prephaser can be placed immediately after the RF pulse, as shown in Figure 30.

7.4.4   Rewinder Gradient

The rewinder gradient area (A_r) is given, using Eq. 22, by:

$$A_r = 1/\gamma\, \delta\, y \tag{43}$$

This gradient pulse can be placed immediately after the acquisition period.

7.4.5   Minimum Sequence Time

Hence, combining Eqs. 40–43, the total sequence time, or minimum repetition time (minTr), of Fig. 30 is:

$$\min Tr = RT + 1.5 \cdot T_s + 3 \cdot RT + \left(T_a - RT\right)/2 + T_a + RT + A_r / G_m$$

$$= \frac{4.5 \cdot G_m}{G_s} + \frac{3}{\gamma \, G_m \Delta z} + \frac{1.5}{\gamma \, G_m \delta x} + \frac{1}{\gamma \, G_m \delta y} \tag{44}$$

Now, evaluating Eq. 44, γ=42.57 kHz/mT (kHz corresponds to the reciprocal of time in ms.) Let the slice thickness and spatial resolution be defined by Δz=7 mm, and $\delta x = \delta y = 1.5$ mm, respectively. Also assume a maximum gradient strength and slew rate of G_m=20 mT/m, and G_s= 100 mT m^{-1} ms^{-1}, respectively. Then Eq. 44 becomes:

$$\min Tr = \frac{4.5 \cdot 20}{100} + \frac{3}{42.57 \cdot 20 \cdot 0.007} + \frac{1.5}{42.57 \cdot 20 \cdot 0.0015} + \frac{1}{42.57 \cdot 20 \cdot 0.0015}$$

$$= 0.9 + 0.503 + 1.175 + 0.783 \tag{45}$$

$$= 3.361 \; ms$$

Note that doubling the maximum gradient strength only reduces the minimum repetition time to 3.031 ms in this example. Also note that for systems with a relatively slow slew rate, a shorter repetition time may be achieved by using less than the maximum gradient strength during the RF pulse and/or the signal acquisition period.

Optimizing a rapid imaging sequence largely involves trading off speed for both patient comfort and safety and image quality. In addition to patient heating due to the RF pulses (Schaefer 1992), there is the possibility of patient nerve stimulation due to the use of high gradient slew rates (Schaefer 1992; Abart et al. 1997). Fortunately these two effects are regulated. A further consideration is the image signal to noise ratio. This is reduced as the readout gradient amplitude is increased due to an increase in the pixel bandwidth.

8   Planar k-Space Sampling Techniques

With the gradient-recalled echo sequence one line of k-space data is collected with each spin excitation. While being more challenging, it is possible to acquire data over a planar region of k-space with each excitation. In a general sense all different types of acquisitions discussed in this section could be termed echo-planar imaging acquisitions. However, the term EPI usually refers to a more specific form of data acquisition, where multiple lines of k-space data are collected without the use of additional RF pulses.

8.1   Echo-Planar Imaging

With EPI the readout gradient is repeatedly applied in a positive and negative manner, and during each transition a small gradient pulse in the phase-encoding direction is applied (Mansfield 1977; see Fig. 31). The effect of this gradient activity is to modulate the spin phase such that the interference of all the spin signals corresponds to the k-space values along a rectilinear path through k-space, for the object being imaged (Fig. 32). Formally; if a vector gradient function is defined by:

$$\mathbf{G}(t) = G_x(t)\mathbf{\hat{x}} + G_y(t)\mathbf{\hat{y}} \tag{46}$$

where $G_x(t)$ and $G_y(t)$ are the time varying x and y gradients, respectively, a k-space vector can be defined as:

$$\mathbf{k}(t) = \int_0^t \mathbf{G}(\tau)\mathbf{d}\tau \tag{47}$$

k(t) represents the k-space trajectory. If x represents a point in the x, y space, the received signal can be written:

$$s(\mathbf{k}(t)) = \iint \rho\,(\mathbf{x}) \cdot \exp(i2\pi\,\mathbf{k}(t) \bullet \mathbf{x})\,d\mathbf{x} \tag{48}$$

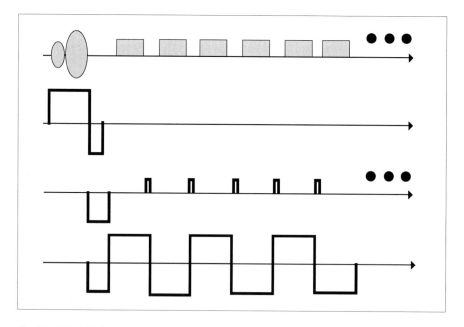

Fig. 31.   The initial portion of an EPI sequence

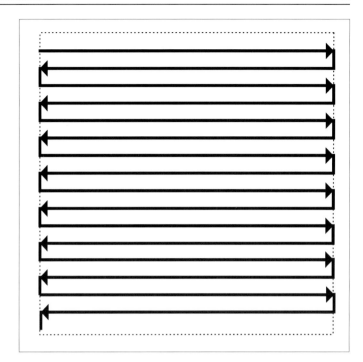

Fig. 32. A rectilinear echo planar k-space trajectory

where ($\cdot$) indicates the scalar product of two vectors. This equation is just a vector representation of a 2D Fourier transform. By varying the gradients in an appropriate manner, the points in k-space (Eq. 47) at which k-space data are acquired can be controlled. Thus the time varying gradients control the trajectory over which the k-space data are acquired.

On the surface it would seem that any trajectory would be as good as any other, provided that k-space is sufficiently well covered. However, due to field inhomogeneities, eddy currents induced by the gradient fields, and imprecision in the control of the time varying gradients fields, some trajectories are better than others. The rectilinear trajectory shown in Figure 32 is the one typically used for EPI. However, even so, the system calibration required with such sequences is an order of magnitude more complex than that necessary to achieve good gradient-recalled echo images.

The advantages of EPI over sequences which only collect a single line of k-space include (a) shorter imaging times as RF pulses do not need to be repeatedly applied, and (b) a longer signal recover time (hence more signal) as the repetition time between RF pulse is larger. However, there are disadvantages, such as (a) a large fat shift, (b) large spatial distortions due to field inhomogeneities, and (c) blurring and signal dropout due to T2* relaxation.

Although it appears from Figure 31 that the oscillating readout section can be repeated indefinitely, this turns out to be misleading. The EPI readout takes time, and this increases with desired image resolution. The problem is that the MR signal decays, and therefore the later k-space lines collected may have very little signal. Thus with single-shot EPI the achievable resolution is limited by T2* relaxation.

The "echo planar" really refers to the readout section of the pulse sequence. Figure 31 is a gradient-recalled echo EPI sequence. It is possible to also have spin-echo EPI sequences. As with the gradient-recalled echo EPI, this is simply a spin-echo sequence with the single k-space line readout replaced by the multiple k-space line EPI readout.

8.1.1   Multishot Echo-Planar Imaging

Single-shot EPI acquires all the k-space data with only one excitation. However, typically the image acquisition matrix is no larger than 128 × 128. To achieve higher resolution, and reduce the image distortion and signal loss due to susceptibility differences, T2 relaxation, and main field inhomogeneities, multishot EPI can be performed (see, for example, McKinnon 1993). Here only a portion of the k-space data is acquired with each excitation (or shot), and the excitations repeated until a full set of data is collected.

The imaging time for an EPI sequence depends basically on the length of the slice selective excitation (Tss) and the time to acquire a number (N) of k-space lines, each of length Tacq:

$$\text{Tepi} = \text{Tss} + \text{N·Tacq} \tag{49}$$

For multishot EPI fewer k-lines are acquired per shot, but more excitations are required. Thus for M shots, the imaging time is:

$$
\begin{aligned}
\text{Tms-epi} \ &= \text{M·(Tss} + \text{N·Tacq/M)} \\
&= \text{M·Tss} + \text{N·Tacq} \\
&= \text{Tepi} + (\text{M}-1)\text{·Tss}
\end{aligned}
\tag{50}
$$

For a 128 × 128 matrix, depending on the gradient system, Tacq and Tss can be about 0.5 ms and 1.5 ms, respectively. For a fractional k-space acquisition 70 lines are acquired. Thus, in this example, the single-shot imaging time is 36.5 ms (= 1.5 + 70 × 0.5). For a four-shot EPI sequence (using this example) the imaging time is only 4.5 ms longer, and the image distortions are reduced by fourfold. The flow sensitivity is also reduced with the number of shots. Hence increasing the number of shots reduces the signal loss in the presence of turbulence.

To avoid ghosting due to k-space phase discontinuities from off resonance signals, two conditions must be met. Firstly the k-space lines must be acquired in an interleaved manner, as illustrated in Figure 33. This is why multishot EPI is sometimes known as interleaved EPI. The second requirement is that the different shots are acquired with an incremental time delay between the RF pulse and the readout. This is known as echo time shifting, and is discussed in McKinnon (1993).

A disadvantage of multishot EPI occurs in situations where T1 weighting is undesirable. Here the potential for reducing the repetition time cannot be utilized, and the imaging time becomes proportional to the number of shots.

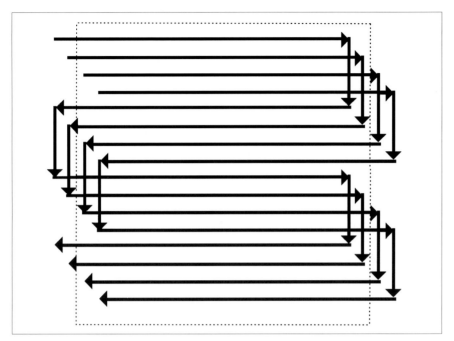

Fig. 33. An set of interleaved echo planar trajectories (drawn offset for clarity)

8.1.2 Asymmetric Echo-Planar Imaging

There are variants of EPI which require less precise system calibration. One of these, asymmetric EPI, collects only data during, say, the positive readout gradient lobe. The, say, negative lobe is used just to traverse back to the other side of k-space (Feinberg et al. 1990). This strategy of only collecting data with either the positive or negative readout gradient lobe is also used for flow compensated EPI sequences. These sequences require more time than conventional EPI; however, their robustness is often a welcome bonus.

8.2 Spiral Imaging

A spiral trajectory (either single or multiple) is the most efficient way of traversing k-space (Meyer et al. 1992). More precisely, a spiral is the fastest trajectory for covering a circular region of k-space for a given set of gradient parameters. Further, spiral trajectories have the convenient feature that the resulting image is very insensitive to the turbulence in flowing blood. Hence vessels appear uniformly intense. On the other hand, image reconstruction of spiral data is more involved than for rectilinear acquired data. Also it is less easy to take advantage of rectangular field of views and fractional k-space concepts to reduce the image acquisition time.

8.3   Fast (Turbo) Spin-Echo Imaging

FSE (sometimes turbo spin echo), or RARE, imaging is similar to EPI in that multiple lines of k-space data are collected with each acquisition (Hennig et al. 1986). The k-space trajectory of a FSE sequence can be derived using an equation similar to Eq. 47.

The addition of the RF refocusing pulses implies that FSE takes longer than EPI. However, they also make the sequence insensitive to field inhomogeneities. Hence there are few problems with spatial distortions, fat shift, or signal dropout.

The FSE sequence is actually quite complicated with respect to its coherence pathways. The main consequence is that the phase of the RF pulses must be carefully controlled.

The addition of the rewinder gradient pulse is necessary for controlling the coherences (see Fig. 34). Nominally the refocusing should be performed with 180° pulses. However, due to the incorporation of many coherences the signal level is only slightly less with, say, 135° pulses.

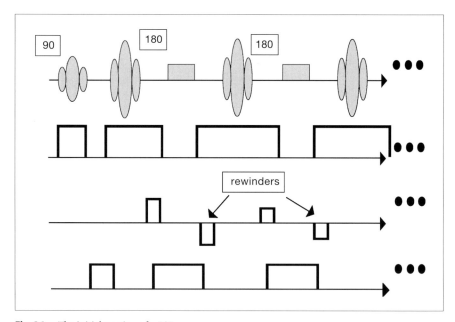

Fig. 34.   The initial portion of a FSE sequence

8.3.1   Multishot and Single-Shot Fast Spin-Echo Imaging

Most clinical FSE imaging is performed in a multishot mode. However, with improvements in gradient performance single-shot FSE has become a useful imaging tool, especially with respect to reducing respiratory artifacts. For single-shot FSE imaging the echo spacing is reduced as much as possible, by using stronger gradient pulses and shorter RF pulses. The RF refocusing pulse angle is also typically reduced to prevent patient heating problems. Note that reducing the refocusing pulse angle does change the image contrast somewhat.

8.3.2   RF Phase Errors

In general the FSE sequence performs very well. However, it is very sensitive to errors in the phase of the RF pulses. The phase of the excitation pulse must be 90° with respect with that of the RF refocusing pulses. Hence applications such as diffusion imaging prove a major challenge. Due to the large motion sensitivity of the diffusion gradients it is practically impossible in vivo to control the tight phase relationships between the excitation and refocusing RF pulses. This leads to regions of signal dropout in the image. However, even here there are techniques for dealing with this, again, by using more specific control of the coherence pathways (Norris et al. 1992). Unfortunately, in this case the price paid is a 50% reduction in signal.

9   Physiological Gating

With ultrafast imaging most abdominal acquisitions can be performed with breath-holding. However, even with EPI it is usually necessary to resort to some form of physiological gating when imaging the heart.

9.1   Prospective and Retrospective Gating

For multiphase cardiac imaging a set of k-lines is repeatedly acquired over one cardiac cycle. Then during the next cardiac cycle the next set of k-lines is acquired. Switching from one set to the next requires a physiological trigger.

For morphological imaging, where imaging the cyclic motion is unimportant, the MR sequence is set to acquire data at a particular phase of the cyclic motion. Again, a physiological trigger followed by a delay period is required to synchronize the acquisition with the motion.

Prospective gating involves pausing the imaging sequence until a trigger signal is detected, repeatedly collecting a set of k-lines and then pausing for the next trigger, etc. This is illustrated in Figure 35. Prospective gating is useful for morphological imaging. However, it has two problems when used to image periodic motion. First, because of the need to wait for a trigger signal, a portion of the cyclic motion is not imaged. The second problem is that there is a variable repetition time between the two acquisitions just before and just after the trigger. As this time varies with variations in the periodicity of the motion, the amount of magnetization recovery due to relaxation mechanisms also varies, which in turn causes variations in the MR signal. This produces image artifacts.

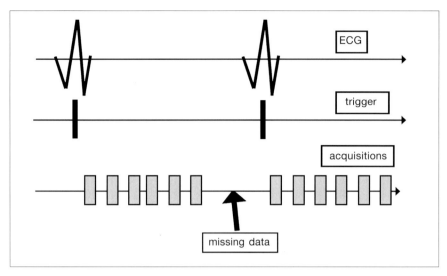

Fig. 35.   Prospective ECG gating

Retrospective gating involves collecting a set of k-lines in a regular manner, as indicated in Fig. 36. Here there is no waiting for a trigger signal. Instead, before each set is acquired, the system checks to see whether a trigger occurred. In the event that a trigger is detected the next set of k-lines is acquired; otherwise the present set is collected again. This strategy eliminates image artifacts due to uneven repetition times, and acquires data over the whole cycle. However, if the motion is irregular, there is a varying number of k-line sets collected each cycle. Postprocessing of the data takes the variable number of sets and interpolates them onto a fixed number, equally spaced throughout the cycle. This is performed before the multiphase image reconstruction is started.

9.2   Segmented K-Space

The previous section mentions that a set of k-lines is repeatedly acquired during a cardiac cycle. Up until a few years ago, however, only one k-line was repeatedly acquired. This meant that an image consisting of 160 phase encodes required 160 heart cycles for its collection. With improved gradient performance it has become possible to collect several different k-lines each cardiac cycle. This form of gated acquisition is called segmented k-space (Atkinson and Edelman 1991).

The main consideration with segmented k-space acquisitions is in determining how many k-lines to collect per set, or more specifically, determining what temporal resolution is required. If, for instance, a temporal resolution of 50 ms is sufficient, and the repetition time is 5 ms, a set would consist of 10 k-lines. Combining segmented k-space with a fractional k-space acquisition would reduce the imaging time in the previous example to about nine heart cycles. Hence the segmented k-space strategy makes breath-held cardiac imaging feasible.

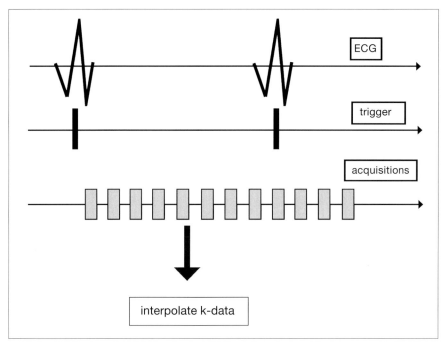

Fig. 36. Retrospective ECG gating

9.3 Navigator Gating and Motion Correction

This is sometimes called respiratory navigator. It is a form of respiratory gating. However, instead of using respiratory bellows to determine the respiratory cycle, an MR experiment is used to determine the position of the diaphragm (Sachs et al. 1994). There are prospective and retrospective forms of navigator gating. The first requires rapid analysis of the navigator measurement, and the result is used to trigger the imaging sequence. The second is largely a postprocessing step. The navigator and imaging measurements are alternated, and then only those k-lines collected within a particular range of diaphragm positions are used to reconstruct the image. It is also possible to use the navigator measurement to reposition the image section in real-time, and hence attempt to follow the motion (Danias et al. 1997).

10   Hardware Considerations

In this section a number of hardware related aspects of fast imaging are examined.

10.1   Gradient Slew Rate

The slew rate is a measure of how rapidly the gradient fields can be switched on or off. The higher the slew rate is, the faster the gradient switching, and hence the shorter the imaging time.

10.1.1   dB/dT Limits

However, there is a catch. Switching gradient fields means that the local magnetic field changes. This rate of magnetic field change is (over the linear region of the gradients) equal to the slew rate times the displacement from isocenter. Generally, magnetic field is denoted by B, hence the rate of change is written dB/dt.

A changing magnetic field induces a current in an electrical conductor. This current is proportional to the area circumscribed by the conductor and the rate of magnetic field change. (Or, more specifically, the amount of magnetic flux passing through the circumscribed area, and the rate of change of the magnetic flux.) While the specific details are complex, the important point is that gradient switching can produce currents which can induce nerve stimulations.

The maximum permitted dB/dt limits are regulated. However, for a given slew rate, the exact value of the magnetic field change depends on the manufacturer's gradient coil configuration. Also note that if more than one gradient field changes at the same time, the total dB/dt is the sum of the contributions from each axis. For instance, if the slew rate is 100 mT m^{-1} ms^{-1} on all three axes, with all three axes being switched at the same time, and dB/dt is to be evaluted at x = 25 cm, y = 25 cm, and z = 25 cm with respect to the gradient isocenter, the total dB/dt (for linear gradients) is:

$$dB/dt = x \, dG_x/dt + y \, dG_y/dt + z \, dGz/dt$$
$$= 0.25 \times 100 + 0.25 \times 100 + 0.25 \times 100 \qquad (51)$$
$$= 75 \text{ mT m}^{-1} \text{ ms}^{-1} \text{ (which is the same as 75 T m}^{-1} \text{ s}^{-1})$$

The interested reader is urged to check the exact regulations with the appropriate regulatory bodies. However, for orientation purposes, 54 T m^{-1} s^{-1} is often assumed as the value for the onset of peripheral nerve stimulation.

10.2   Gradient Strength

Generally, gradient pulses are designed with a specific area. Hence the stronger the gradient is, the shorter the sequence time. However, stronger gradient fields also bring problems.

10.2.1 Maxwell Terms

Gradient fields are generally assumed to produce a z-directed magnetic field, with linear gradients in the x, y, or z directions. However, according to Maxwell's electromagnetic field equations, it is impossible to have a nonconstant magnetic field orientated in a constant direction (see, for example, Jackson 1975). The gradients of the x and y directed components are actually similar in magnitude to the gradient of the z component. Consider just a z gradient field (G_z); Maxwell's equations indicate that the total (vector) magnetic field is:

$$\mathbf{B_T} = \begin{bmatrix} B_x \\ B_y \\ B_z \end{bmatrix} = \begin{bmatrix} -xG_z/2 \\ -yG_z/2 \\ B_0 + zG_z \end{bmatrix} \tag{52}$$

Hence the magnitude of the total field, B, is:

$$B = \sqrt{B_x^2 + B_y^2 + B_z^2}$$
$$\approx B_0 + zG_z + \left(x^2 + y^2\right)\frac{G_z^2}{8B_0} \tag{53}$$

The third term in Eq. 53 represents an addition to the spin precession frequency. Notice that it depends on the square of the gradient field. Thus the additional precession frequency does not change sign if the gradient is reversed. This can cause some image artifacts (Norris and Hutchinson 1990).

The Maxwell terms (or the additional gradient field components) can cause velocity estimation errors for off-isocenter phase contrast imaging and additional spatial distortions for EPI. Many of these can be corrected, however (Bernstein et al. 1997).

10.2.2 Eddy Currents

Gradient switching can induce eddy currents which in turn produce additional magnetic fields. These can result in spatial distortions, particularly with EPI. The rate of increase in eddy current is proportional to the gradient slew rate. The total amount of eddy current produced (for time constants longer than the switching time) is the product of slew rate and the amount of time the gradient is slewing (or the switching time). Thus the total eddy current is proportional simply to the maximum gradient amplitude reached. In other words, to a good approximation, the eddy current fields are independent of slew rate, even though the gradient switching is their primary cause.

10.3   Gradient Limited Imaging Speed

In order to reduce imaging time gradient slew rate and/or maximum amplitude can be increased. However, merely doubling one or the other provides surprisingly little improvement. This situation can nevertheless be appreciated when one considers that the only certain way of doubling the gradient-limited imaging speed is simultaneously to double the maximum gradient amplitude and increase the gradient slew rate by a factor of four. This operation retains the gradient pulse areas while halving the time scale. In the past few years most manufacturers have actually done just this. Several years ago the standard high-end systems had a maximum gradient strength of about 10 mT m^{-1} and a slew rate of about 20 mT m^{-1} ms^{-1}. Now the maximum gradient is around 20 mT m^{-1}, with a slew rate of about 80 mT m^{-1} ms^{-1}. Hence the gradient limited imaging speed has been doubled. Due to the dB/dt issues mentioned above it is difficult to envisage this being repeated without using small dedicated gradient coils.

10.4   Sampling Bandwidth

This is another hardware term which is very much part of the fast imaging vocabulary. For ultrafast imaging the sampling bandwidth needs to be higher than that generally used for more conventional clinical imaging. Its easy to appreciate why. With a 20-kHz sampling rate it takes 12.8 ms to acquire 256 samples. At a 200 kHz sampling rate only 1.28 ms are necessary. The penalty, as discussed in Sect. 4.2, is the reduced signal to noise ratio.

The maximum sampling bandwidth of an MR system places limits on the field of view that can be acquired, with the readout gradient using the maximum gradient strength. The relationship is given by Eq. 25. As an example, if the maximum gradient strength is 20 mT/m, and the maximum sampling rate is 200 kHz (full bandwidth), the maximum field of view with full utilization of the gradients is:

$$FOV = 200 \text{ kHz} / (42.57 \text{ kHz/mT} \times 20 \text{ mT/m})$$
$$= 0.23 \text{ m (or 23 cm)} \tag{54}$$

This does not mean that 23 cm is the maximum field of view, but rather that for fields of view larger than 23 cm the readout gradient must be less than the maximum gradient strength, which could increase the minimum sequence time.

A further issue related to sampling bandwidth is that digital receivers typically have discrete sampling bandwidths. This can seem restrictive; however, it need not impinge on imaging performance. The key parameter with respect to image quality is pixel bandwidth. Hence for a desired pixel bandwidth (bw_p), pixel resolution (Δx), and a minimum field of view (FOV_{min}), the minimum sampling frequence (f_{min}) is:

$$f_{min} = bw_p \ FOV_{min} / \Delta x \tag{55}$$

If f_{next} is the next highest discrete sampling frequency, the measurement can be performed with both Δx and FOV increased by the factor f_{next}/f_{min}. This does not change the signal to noise ratio or the data acquisition period. The only drawback is that the number of samples and the field of view are larger than necessary. However, the field of view can be truncated automatically after the image reconstruction.

References

Abart J, Eberhardt K, Fischer H, Huk W, Richter E, Schmitt F, Storch T, Zeitler E (1997) Peripheral nerve stimulation by time-varying magnetic fields. J Compt Assist Tomogr 21:532–538

Atkinson DJ, Edelman RR (1991) Cine-angiography of the heart in a single breath-hold with a segmented turboFLASH sequence. Radiology 178:357–360

Bernstein MA, Zhou X, King KF, Ganin A, Pelc NJ, Glover GH (1997) Shading artifacts in phase contrast angiography induced by Maxwell terms: analysis and correction. Int Soc Magn Reson Med, annual meeting abstracts, p 110

Bracewell RN (1978) The Fourier transform and its applications. McGraw-Hill, New York

Danias PG, McConnell MV, Khasgiwala VC, Chuang ML, Edelman RR, Manning WJ (1997) Prospective navigator correction of image position for coronary MR. Radiology 203:733–736

Du YP, Parker DL, Davis WL, Cao G (1994) Reduction of partial volume artifacts with zerofilled interpolation in 3D MRA. J Magn Reson Imag 4:733–741

Feinberg DA, Turner R, Kakab PD, von Kienlin M (1990) Echo-planar imaging with asymmetric gradient modulation and inner-volume excitation. Magn Reson Med 13:162–169

Hennig J (1988) Multiecho imaging sequences with low refocusing flip angles. J Magn Reson 78:397–407

Hennig J, Nauerth A, Friedburg H (1986) RARE imaging: a fast imaging method for clinical MR. Magn Reson Med 3:823–833

Jackson JD (1975) Classical electromagnetics. Wiley, New York

Ljunggren S (1983) A simple graphical representation of Fourier based imaging methods. J Magn Reson 54:338–343

Mansfield P (1977) Multiplanar image formation using NMR spin echoes. J Phys C Solid State Phys 10:L55–l58

McKinnon GC (1993) Ultrafast interleaved gradient echo-planar imaging on a standard scanner. Magn Reson Med 30:609–616

Meyer CH, Hu BS, Nishimura DG, Macovski A (1992) Fast spiral coronary artery imaging. Magn Reson Med 28:202–213

Morse PM, Feshbach H (1953) Methods of theoretical physics. McGraw-Hill, New York

Norris DG, Hutchison JMS (1990) Concomitant magnetic field gradients and their effects on imaging at low magnetic field strengths. Magn Reson Imaging 8:33–37

Norris DG, Bornert P, Reese T, Leibfritz D (1992) On the application of the ultra-fast RARE experiments. Magn Reson Med 27:142–164

Sachs TS, Meyer CH, Hu BS, Kohli J, Nishimura DG (1994) Real-time motion detection in spiral MRI using navigators. Magn Reson Med 32:639–645

Schaefer DJ (1992) Dosimetry and effects of MR exposure to RF and switched magnetic fields. Ann NY Acad Sci 649:225–236

Slichter CP (1980) Principles of magnetic resonance. Springer, Berlin Heidelberg New York

Twieg DB (1983) The k-trajectory formulation of the NMR imaging process with applications in analysis and synthesis of imaging methods. Med Phys 10:610–621

van der Meulen P (1988) Fast field echo imaging: an overview and contrast calculations. Magn Reson Imaging 6:355–368

Zur Y, Wood ML, Neuringer LJ (1991) Spoiling of transverse magnetization in steady-state sequences. Magn Reson Med 21:251–263

2 Ultrafast Magnetic Resonance Imaging of the Brain and Spine

I. Berry, J.-P. Ranjeva, P. Duthil, and C. Manelfe

1 Morphology

Ultrafast MR imaging strategies are useful in the assessment of neurological morphology as well as function. Reflecting inevitable trade-offs between spatial resolution and data acquisition speed, ultrafast MRI is, however, limited in its ability to explore morphology. Obvious indications include the fast examination of a restless patient with half k-space sampling, which can serve as a screening procedure. Fetal brain imaging might be considered another, more original application of ultrafast brain imaging. Limitations of the ultrafast MRI assessment of cerebral morphology become apparent, however, when detection of multiple sclerosis plaques is considered. In the spine, ultrafast imaging permits the evaluation of dynamic motion processes.

1.1 Magnetic Resonance Imaging of the Fetal Brain with HASTE

Fetal MRI should be considered when a brain malformation is suspected based on an ultrasound examination. Imaging must be sufficiently rapid to avoid corrupting artifacts from fetal or maternal motion. This can be accomplished even without sedation or curarization with the HASTE technique (half-Fourier acquisition single-shot turbo spin echo) (Fig. 1). Morphologic evaluation of the fetal brain becomes meaningful beyond a gestational age of 25 weeks. The principal indications for such an examination are ventricular dilatation with suspicion of agenesis of the commissures such as callosal agenesis, posterior fossa malformations, microcephaly, macrocephaly, and craniostenosis.

Short examination times make fetal MRI examinations easy to perform: a series of five images in each of the three orthogonal planes can be acquired in less than 1 min. Reflecting better contrast and spatial resolution, fetal brain MRI offers a diagnostic potential well beyond that associated with ultrasound (D'Ercole et al. 1993; Wenstrom et al. 1991). Concerns regarding MRI-associated harmful side-effects on placental or fetal development, particularly development of the brain, have been thoroughly addressed. To date, neither magnetic field strength nor radiofrequency power nor the intense sound of the magnetic field gradient switching have been associated with any adverse effect.

We would like to acknowledge M. Clanet, M.D., and A. Sevely, M.D., for their kind cooperation.

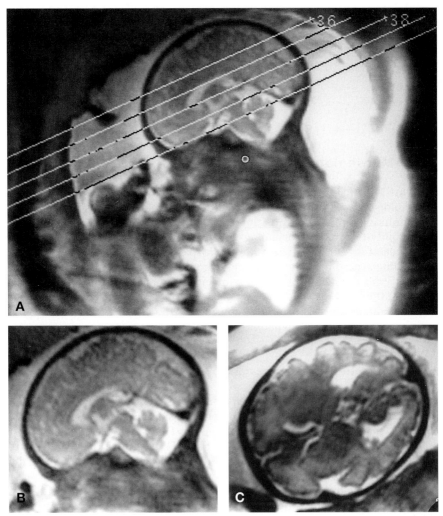

Fig. 1A–C. Fetal MRI. The HASTE sequence samples only half of the Fourier space in a single shot. Asymmetry of sampling is minimized by an initial collection of the first seven lines, followed by the collection of the central lines and the rest of the half Fourier plane. Each echo is obtained after refocussing with an intense radiofrequency pulse 1.28 ms in duration. The interval between each echo and the next is 10.92 ms. The longer echo time is 1200 ms, but the effective TE for contrast weighting is 87 ms, that is, immediately after the first seven-line collection. This moderates the T2 weighting. The matrix size is 240 ×256 with a field of view of 400 × 400 mm. Slice thickness is 5 mm. Five slices are sampled in each direction; each series is collected over 10 s. The entire examination takes 1 min. MRI was performed for the assessment of minor ventriculomegaly and delay of femoral growth in a 36-week-old fetus with normal caryotype. Corpus callosus agenesis was suspected and ruled out on this examination. (**A**) Sagittal view allowed centering axial topogram of five axial slices through the brain of the fetus. (**B**) Midline sagittal view confirms the presence of the corpus callosum and integrity of brain structures. (**C**) Axial plane of the brain shows ventriculomegaly, which appears bilateral and symmetrical.

Additionally, more than 10 years of experience with imaging pregnant women has failed to reveal any harmful effects (Colletti et al. 1994; Kanal 1994).

Initial MRI protocols involved paralyzing the fetus by injecting curare in the umbilical vein subsequent to obtaining a fetal blood sample required for caryotyping. With this technique excellent MR imaging quality could be achieved even with conventional sequences (Girard et al. 1995). Neuronal migration could be studied in vivo (Girard and Raybaud 1992). For ethical reasons this invasive procedure was restricted to fetuses in which umbilical vein blood samples were required for other reasons (Girard et al. 1995).

In an attempt to overcome motion artifacts without curarization, echo-planar imaging (EPI) was tested (Baker et al. 1995). The results were disappointing as image quality was adversely affected by magnetic susceptibility and chemical shift artifacts. While image quality was sufficient to provide fetal biometric data, an accurate morphological assessment of the brain was not possible (Garden et al. 1991).

Somewhat slower than EPI, the HASTE technique provides adequate image quality while limiting artifacts from fetal motion and maternal breathing. Despite the considerable gradient permutation sound upon sequence initialization, the images are only minimally affected by fetal motion. The HASTE technique renders T2-weighted images which depict myelinization to good advantage (Revel et al. 1992).

1.2   Ultrafast Multiple Sclerosis (MS) Plaque Imaging

The FLAIR (fluid-attenuated inversion-recovery) sequence has been shown to be of particular value in the assessment of the periventricular region as it renders CSF signal within the ventricles dark, whilst maintaining a high sensitivity for intraparenchymal fluid. Acquisition times are long, however (de Coene et al. 1992). Data acquisition times can be considerably shortened if several echoes are obtained and rearranged in Fourier space (turbo-FLAIR). By integrating the HASTE sequence design into FLAIR (FLAIR-HASTE), the acquisition can be further accelerated while maintaining FLAIR's inherent sensitivity to fluid attenuations. This can facilitate visualization of multiple sclerosis (MS) plaques in the periventricular and subcortical white matter. FLAIR-HASTE shows MS lesions as containing hyperintense signal, which can be easily differentiated from the dark signal characteristic of CSF in FLAIR sequences. It was thought that this type of sequence could serve as a screening procedure for MS because of the extremely short acquisition time. The high magnetization transfer effect and low rate of susceptibility artifacts were also considered beneficial.

Despite initial enthusiasm, limitations of HASTE soon became apparent (Fig. 2). For coverage of the entire brain, 13 sections, each collected over 3.7 s, are acquired. Image quality, however, was found to be inferior to that of turbo-FLAIR imaging with an acquisition time of 4.24 min. Thus, for applications warranting the highest image quality, such as MS plaque imaging, HASTE-FLAIR should not be considered the first choice.

The use of EPI acquisition strategies results in a further shortening of imaging times (Simonson et al. 1994). Data collection for a single section (matrix 256 × 128) is possible in under 100 ms. Compromises with regard to image quality, induced by magnetic susceptibility artifacts at the skull base and sinus interfaces limit the diagnostic confidence in the identification of MS lesions. In a blinded comparison of T2-weighted spin echo and EPI-FLAIR the diagnostic quality of T2-weighted spin-echo images was found to be superior except in the presence of motion artifacts.

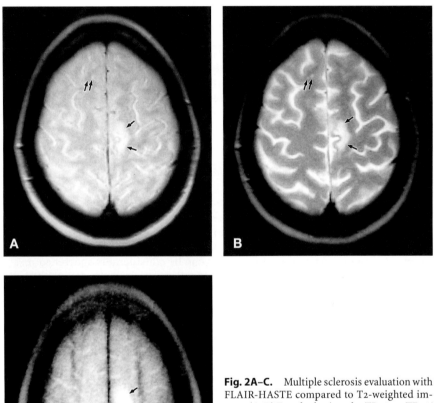

Fig. 2A–C. Multiple sclerosis evaluation with FLAIR-HASTE compared to T2-weighted images. (**A, B**) Fast dual spin-echo TR 3800, TE 16/98 ms, rectangular field of view and matrix (224 × 256), acquisition time 2.56 min. Subcortical MS lesions (*arrows*). (**C**) HASTE-FLAIR sequence with effective TE 87 ms, TI 2500 ms, rectangular field of view (219 × 250), rectangular matrix (240 halved × 256), 1 excitation, acquisition time 3.7 s for a single slice (2.29 min for 13 slices). The largest lesion is seen on HASTE imaging, but the two smaller plaques are not visualized

1.3   Dynamic Evaluation of Cervical Spine Motion

Dynamic evaluation of the cervical spine has been shown to be useful in patients with rheumatoid arthritis, post-traumatic cervical sprain, and degenerative disease. Many abnormalities are best seen in a stress position; some are not visible at all in the neutral resting position of the neck. The latter has been shown to be particularly true for spondylolisthesis, retrolisthesis, and anterior atlanto-axoid subluxations. While functional X-ray studies are of great help in such conditions, they are limited to demonstrating the bony constituents. Intervertebral disks and ligaments cannot be visualized, nor can the functional reserve of the CSF space be assessed. Dynamic cervical myelography was thus used for many years to evaluate the caliber of the spinal canal.

Dynamic MRI of the spine provides functional data in conjunction with a thorough analysis of spinal morphology. With rapid sagittal HASTE MRI, several positions of the cervical spine can be imaged and reproduced in a cine mode (Guyer et al. 1992). Extension of the cervical spine reveals narrowing of the posterior subarachnoid space due to thickening and bulging of the flaval ligament, which is related to decreased elasticity. Compression of the subarachnoid space or even the spinal cord is well assessed on the T2-weighted myelographic HASTE sequences.

Short imaging times of 2 min or less make HASTE well suited for imaging the spine in different positions (Fig. 3). The pronounced myelographic effect adequately depicts the anterior and posterior subarachnoid spaces and permits measurement of the cervical spine in every position. Contrast-enhanced T1-weighted images are also reliable for assessing the cord parenchyma. Pathologic processes such as posterior disk herniations or protrusions are well depicted, as are protrusions of the posterior longitudinal ligaments and bulging of the flaval ligaments. Narrow canals can be properly assessed. At the level of the craniocervical junction, the location and volume of inflammatory pannus and the consequences of horizontal or vertical anterior atlanto-axoid luxation can be evaluated. Limitations of this technique are related to poor visualization of the anterior atlanto-axoid articulation, lack of pannus tissue characterization, and poor definition of the signal within the intervertebral disks.

2   Function

2.1   Functional MRI

Understanding brain function remains a fascinating challenge. A considerable amount of energy has been expended in this endeavor. Thus the diseased brain has been extensively studied post mortem in an attempt to explore the mechanisms underlying brain function. The controversy over the interaction between reason and emotion has been ongoing for centuries (Damasio 1994). Further input into this debate has been provided by the possibility of viewing and studying pathologic cerebral function in living patients using neuroradiological tools (Moseley 1995) and, more recently, of showing specifically which areas

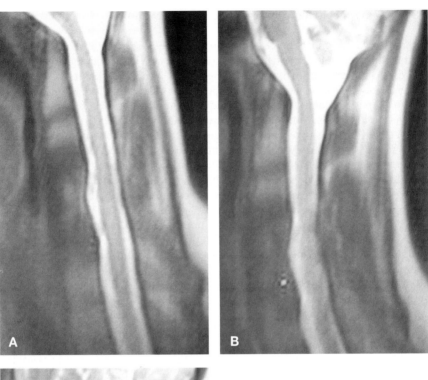

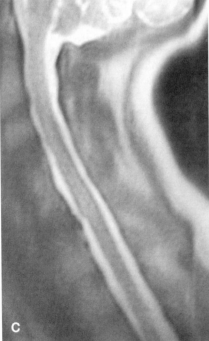

Fig. 3A–C. Postoperative control for tear-drop fracture of C5 in a 22-year-old woman. Mono-slice (5 mm thick) HASTE imaging in multiple positions of the cervical spine, of which three are selected: flexion (**A**), neutral (**B**), and extension (**C**). T2 weighting is ensured by an effective TE of 87 ms and a flip angle of 12°. Resolution parameters include a field of view of 250 × 250 mm in a data matrix size of 240 (halved) × 256. Acquisition time amounts to 2 s per acquired slice. Posterior osteosynthesis of C4–C6 produces a flexion with a higher rotation center than normal, centered at the level C3–C4. Dynamic MR cervical myelography rules out cord compression because the cerebrospinal white layer of fluid is maintained in every position

of the brain are involved in the performance of various tasks (Potchen and Potchen 1991).

Prior to recognizing MRI's capabilities regarding the exploration of cerebral function and activation pathways, functional brain studies were based upon radioactive tracers of cerebral blood flow (Turner 1994; Cohen and Bookheimer 1994; Sergent 1994; Sawle 1995). Building upon this experience, initial MRI experiments used contrast agent boluses (Belliveau et al. 1990, 1991) to assess brain perfusion. Subsequently the signal modifications based on local variations of deoxyhemoglobin in red blood cells were discovered and used to identify regions within the brain involved in the performance of specific tasks: the term functional MRI (fMRI) became associated with this technique (Turner et al. 1993; Kwong et al. 1992; Bandettini et al. 1992; Ogawa et al. 1992). Subsequent research pursued two avenues: fundamental work, attempting to better characterize the origin of the observed signal modulations, and applied work by multidisciplinary groups adapting neuropsychological tests to MRI. The latter approach gave rise to two distinct fields: purely cognitive research, usually performed at high magnetic fields for higher sensitivity (Ugurbil et al. 1993; Turner and Jezzard 1994), and a more clinically focused utilization of fMRI directly deriving from the results of the cognitive research (Turner et al. 1993). With MRI becoming increasingly available throughout the world, clinical use of fMRI soon became widespread. This developement was aided by the fact that most fMRI applications, particularly those identifying the primary cortex areas, could be immediately adapted for clinical imagers at 1.5 T operating with conventional hardware (Turner et al. 1993; Connely et al. 1993; Constable et al. 1993; Schad et al. 1993; Thompson et al. 1994). Therefore, a large multicenter evaluation of clinical fMRI using both conventional systems and systems with high-performance EPI hardware is now under way.

2.1.1 Principle of BOLD Imaging

The signal enhancement observed in brain activation studies reflects a decrease in deoxyhemoglobin concentration in the microvasculature resulting from a local increase of blood oxygenation during cerebral tissue activation. The induced increase in magnetic homogeneity results in an MR signal change which is referred to as the BOLD (blood oxygen level-dependent) effect. Functional and structural information can be superimposed on the same image. Comparison of fMRI brain mapping with positron emission tomography (PET), coupled with improvements in data acquisition strategies, providing submillimeter pixel resolution, as well as in post-processing methods, have considerably enhanced the clinical acceptance of fMRI.

The mechanism involved in the signal change is best thought of as a complex cascade of hemodynamic alterations. The BOLD contrast is determined by the deoxyhemoglobin content in the venous compartment of the capillary bed as well as in larger venous structures. The location of the signal may therefore differ from the actual location of the activated cortex. Indeed, the signal may be derived mostly from large epidural veins far distant from the territory they drain.

This was proven by means of high-resolution fMRI correlated with the venous phase of digital angiography (Thompson et al. 1994; Frahm et al. 1993). MR angiography performed at rest and during activation to evaluate the modification of the veins revealed that large venous structures are apparently highly responsive to activation. Nevertheless, it seems that smaller veins such as the subpial veins, and also the veins located between cortical cell layers, are involved as well. Modelling studies have been undertaken to help elucidate the role of the different venous structures and blood flow-associated time of flight effects, as well as the influence of technique (gradient-echo EPI vs spin-echo EPI) and choice of individual imaging parameters (Menon et al. 1993).

2.1.2   Practical Aspects of fMRI

Clinical fMRI is possible both on high-performance systems with EPI capabilities and on conventional systems using gradient-echo techniques. It is essentially based on the direct comparison with protocols established in normal subjects. The clinically most relevant results are reviewed in the following paragraphs.

Functional MRI protocols are still in the developmental stage. They are designed for specific activation tasks, with particular consideration of the required imaging time, data acquisition repetition rate, and the topography of the region concerned. After positioning the patient comfortably to keep motion to a minimum, anatomical images are obtained. Following adjustment of field homogeneity, functional data are collected with a technique emphasizing magnetic susceptibility in conjunction with a high signal-to-noise ratio. Indeed, the most relevant problem of BOLD contrast is the low amplitude of the phenomenon.

On standard imagers, a mono-slice gradient-echo sequence may be chosen with a TE on the order of 40–60 ms, the shortest repetition time possible (i.e., 20–50 ms) and a small flip angle ranging between 10° and 40°. The acquisition bandwidth should be kept narrow in order to increase the signal-to-noise ratio. Slice thickness, matrix size, and field of view are adjusted to achieve a compromise between the demands for sufficient signal (large voxels) and spatial resolution (small voxels). Sequences of images covering alternating periods of rest and stimulation are obtained with a high proportion of imaging time (on the order of 80%)(Connely et al. 1993; Constable et al. 1993; Schad et al. 1993; Thompson et al. 1994).

On imagers equipped with gradients permitting the use of EPI data collection strategies, the proportion of actual data acquisition time within the entire duration of the examination is much smaller. The parameters are also set for magnetic susceptibility weighting of the acquired images. At clinical magnetic fields FID-EPI is employed with, for example, an effective TE of 60 ms, a flip angle of 90°, and a wider bandwidth of around 800 Hz/pixel (Fig. 4). If a single slice is repeated every 3 s, the effective imaging time amounts to merely 4% of the total examination time. Systems now allow multislice EPI acquisitions to be repeated for long series of measurements. Of course, considerable

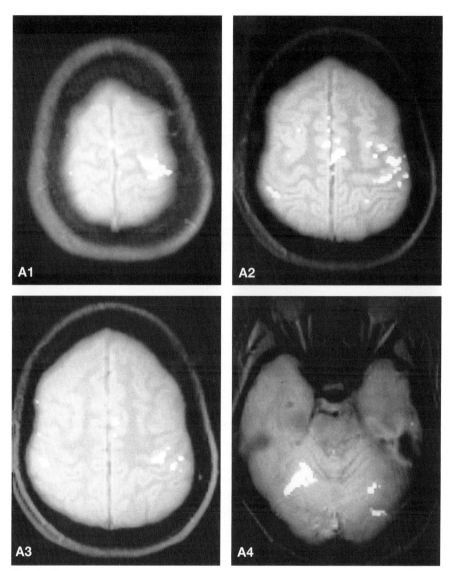

Fig. 4A–C

computing power and storage space is required to handle the enormous data volume generated within a very short time. By covering a larger volume, multislice fMRI acquisitions vastly extend the screening of activated areas at the cost of increasing the proportion of data collection time. Thus, for the assessment of ten sections acquired every 3 s, the effective imaging time amounts to 50% of the total examination time.

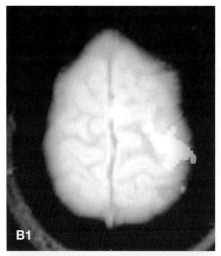
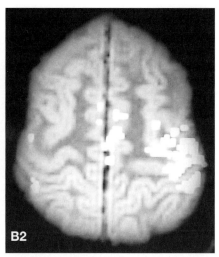

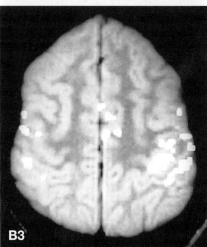

Fig. 4A–C. Motor fMRI in a right-handed normal volunteer. 1.5 T FID-EPI with an effective TE of 60 ms, a flip angle of 90°, and a wide bandwidth (800 Hz/pixel). A 200 × 200 mm field of view is combined with a 64 × 64 matrix. Ten contiguous sections, 5 mm thick, are selected. Eight slices traverse the supratentorial region, two the cerebellum. Images are acquired every 3 s during periods of rest and activation, each lasting 30 s. The activation cycle is repeated four times. The proportion of imaging time is 50%. (A) The task of the right-hand finger opposite the thumb at 1 Hz. Activation of the left primary motor cortex (A1), premotor cortex, and supplementary motor area interhemispherically (A2, A3), as well as the dentate nucleus of the cerebellum are shown (A4). (B) The task of the right-hand finger opposite the thumb at 2 Hz. Greater activation is induced with this more complex task, which involves more of the supplementary motor area and premotor cortex (B2, B3) than the first task (A). (C) The task of the left-hand finger opposite the thumb at 1 Hz. Greater activation is produced with the nondominant hand, even in performing a simple task

The design of the neuropsychological test is referred to as the paradigm. Images are collected in the sequential mode during periods of various activation states. Comparison of the resting state to that during accomplishment of a simple task identifies areas which are specifically involved in primary task processing. Additionally, images of different phases of similar types of activation may be analyzed to reveal specific areas involved in associative processing (e.g., tone and word processing tasks to suppress the contribution of the primary

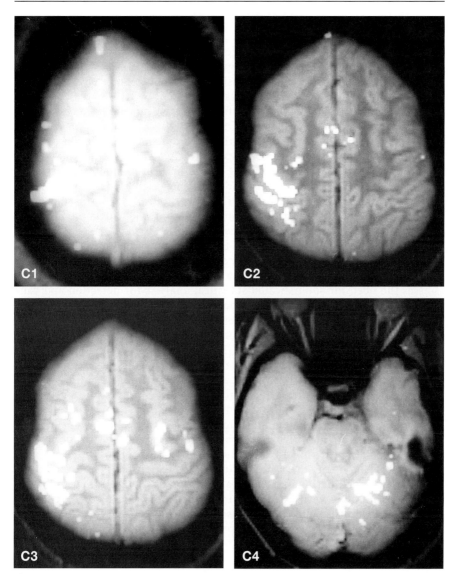

Fig. 4C

auditory contribution; Berry et al. 1995). Although theoretically the duration of task performance need not be very long for the hemodynamic changes to occur (changes in deoxyhemoglobin take place within a few seconds), exposure to the particular stimulus should last at least 30 s in order to allow the patients to mentally settle into each phase. To permit validation of brain activation, fMRI sequences are generally repeated several times (verifying whether changes in signal are consistently coherent with the pattern of rest and activation). This is possible without any problem as the BOLD technique is fully reversible and repeatable with no need for injection of contrast. This must be considered a great advantage over methods employing radioactive material injections such as PET or SPECT (single photon emission computed tomography) which are limited in the number of possible activation phases.

Particularly if EPI data collection strategies are available, fMRI is characterized by high temporal resolution. The BOLD effect takes a few seconds to occur. Signal variations over time reproduce a dynamic stimulation pattern. This allows for the study of the behavior of activated areas over time. Some responses, particularly those requiring a high level of mental concentration, have been shown to decrease over time. Another possibility is to compare response rise times in different locations (Binder et al. 1993). Furthermore, the differential study of the repetition of an activation can elucidate the influence of response habituation to a specific task.

The postprocessing phase is crucial to the success of the fMRI experiment. Indeed, functional SI changes are very subtle ranging between 15–25% in primary activated cortex, and less than 2% in associative activations. This stresses the need for sophisticated statistical analysis for detection and validation of the responding areas (Friston et al. 1995). The greatest danger to a successful fMRI study is patient motion. It is therefore crucial to control patient movement during data acquisition. The problem is compounded by the fact that patients imaged by means of fMRI are part of a population in whom involuntary movements are highly likely to occur during task performance. Cerebral pathologies may even induce synkinesia. Realignment algorithms have thus been developed and found to be useful in various clinical protocols (Wood et al. 1992). Fusion of anatomic and functional datasets following reorientation is also one of the most important postprocessing steps in clinical fMRI, just as in cognitive research. It allows for fine localization of regions of activation, taking advantage of the high spatial resolution of anatomic MRI. This opens the way for single-case experiments and individual identification of functional variations. Additionally, longitudinal follow-up studies are possible with fMRI, requiring special attention to correct slice positioning and threshold setting for significance analysis. Nevertheless, the intrinsic variability of magnetic susceptibility over time remains to be assessed in more detail.

2.1.3 *Normal Results of Brain Activations*

2.1.3.1 Cortical Activations in Normal Subjects

Performance of a task activates regions of the cerebral cortex compared to the rest condition. For example, voluntary movements of one hand activate the contralateral precentral cortex; visualization of a flashing light activates the calcarine cortex in the occipital lobe; and audition activates the superior temporal gyrus. These are primary functions whose corresponding area of activation can readily be detected by both standard GRE- and EPI techniques on an individual basis. On the other hand, activated areas which correspond to lesser increases in blood flow are more difficult to detect on examinations performed on single individuals.

Visual Cortex.   Recent reports comparing character search and checkerboard stimulation tasks (Schneider et al. 1994) have detailed the topography of the human primary visual cortex with a spatial resolution of 1.4 mm (Engel et al. 1994). This work enabled the drawing of retinotopic maps: as the stimulus moved from the fovea to the periphery, the location of responding neurons varied from posterior to anterior portions of the calcarine sulcus. The time course of the responses also varied, depending on the location: activation of peripheral locations were delayed relative to foveal locations, resulting in delayed neural activity in the anterior portion of the calcarine sulcus relative to the posterior calcarine sulcus.

Motor Cortex.   Motor-related activity occurs in several areas of the cortex in response to real or imagined movements. Primary cortices have been accurately identified following specific activation by fMRI. Somatotopic maps of the contralateral primary motor cortex can been rendered after repetitive movements of the fingers (Fig. 4), elbow, and toes in healthy individuals (Rao et al. 1995). Recently, Tyska et al. (1994) identified separate foci of activation permitting localization of the region of the supplementary motor area and the adjacent cingulate cortex. The findings matched the results known from PET and SPECT, stressing the role of such zones in the ideation and initiation of movement (Deiber et al. 1991; Sabatini et al. 1993). Rao et al. (1993) carefully studied voluntary motor control. They found additional activation in the supplementary motor area, the premotor cortex bilaterally, and the contralateral somatosensory cortex during complex self-paced movements, compared to a response limited to the contralateral primary motor cortex in simple self-paced movements. Imagined complex movements activated the supplementary motor area and, to a lesser degree, the premotor cortex.

Sensory Cortex.   The somatosensory cortex was identified by periodic tactile stimulation of the palm of the right hand (Hammeke et al. 1994). Temporally correlated activation was identified in the peri-rolandic region. On the sagittal images, the areas of greatest increase in signal occurred 14–34 mm mesial to the most lateral edge of the temporal surface, which is the correct location expected from stimulation of the hand, on the sensory homunculus. Signal occurred not only on the brain surface but also in the central sulcus, including both the posterior bank of the precentral gyrus and the anterior bank of the postcentral gyrus.

Auditory Cortex and Language Organization.   Signal alterations in the superior temporal gyrus and superior temporal sulcus were observed bilaterally when normal subjects listened to auditory stimuli including nonspeech noise, meaningless speech sounds, single words, and narrative text (Binder et al. 1994). Speech stimuli were associated with significantly more widespread signal changes than was the noise stimulus. No consistent differences were observed among responses to different speech stimuli.

The strategy of contrast between association tasks with similar primary input is particularly well suited to auditory experiments. In such experiments the low proportion of imaging time required by EPI is of particular interest because of the lesser interference with the paradigm (McCarthy et al. 1993).

Gender differences in the functional organization of the brain for language have recently been demonstrated by fMRI. The language function is highly lateralized in males but represented in both cerebral hemispheres in females. Phonological processing was lateralized to the left inferior frontal gyrus in males and spread more diffusely to both left and right inferior frontal gyrus in females (Shaywitz et al. 1995a). Additionally, phonological processing was shown to engage the anterior left temporal lobe. Semantic processing, on the other hand, also involved the left posterior temporal region (Shaywitz et al. 1995b). These results concur with those of other fMRI experiments (Berry et al. 1995) and corroborate PET findings (Demonet et al. 1992).

Memory.   Activation of the middle and inferior frontal gyri was observed in individual subjects during performance of a nonspatial working memory task, namely, observing sequences of letters and responding whenever a letter repeated with exactly one nonidentical letter intervening (Cohen et al. 1994). The control task in this association task study was the comparison of sequences of letters to identify any occurrence of a single, prespecified target letter.

2.1.3.2 Central Activations in Normal Subjects
Initially, areas of activation were depicted in the cortex. More recently, the improved spatial resolution of MRI has allowed the identification of deep structure involvement in the performance of tasks during photic stimulation Kleinschmidt et al. (1994) detected simultaneous signal changes in the lateral geniculate nucleus and in the primary visual cortex. They were the first to demonstrate thalamocortical interaction in the primary visual pathway of the intact human brain.

In the motor system, the activation of putamen and globus pallidus was identified during rapid supination and pronation of the contralateral hand (Bucher et al. 1995). In the cognitive sphere, bilateral involvement of the dentate nucleus of the cerebellum was shown in subjects attempting to solve a pegboard puzzle. This experiment confirmed involvement of the cerebellum not only in the control of movement but also in cognitive functions (Kim et al. 1994).

2.1.4   Clinical Applications of fMRI of the Brain

Among the earliest clinical applications aimed at the evaluation of cerebral pathology, dysfunctional activation of the dentate nuclei, the left inferior olivary nucleus, and the left red nucleus was demonstrated in a patient with palatal myoclonus (Boecker 1994). Initial clinical reports mostly concerned patients with brain tumors.

2.1.4.1 Presurgical Localization of Functional Areas

Pre-operative functional mapping of the cerebral cortex with fMRI has been shown to correlate well with the Wada test involving the intracarotid injection of amobarbital, as well as with intraoperative electrocortical stimulation mapping in patients with epilepsy referred for temporal lobectomy (Hammeke et al. 1994). In fact fMRI has been validated thoroughly by intraoperative cortical mapping including direct cortical stimulation and/or sensory evoked potential recording (Mueller et al. 1996; Jack et al. 1994; Chapman et al. 1995). In all cases, results of cortical function mapping with invasive techniques matched those obtained with fMRI. Sensory cortex activation was identified in the perirolandic area despite the fact that edema from a temporal lobe tumor caused a superior shift in the sylvian fissure of approximately 1 cm. Sensorimotor cortex mapping was performed in two patients with intractable, simple partial motor seizures due to tumors located in or near this cortex.

Soon, other investigators confirmed the ability of fMRI to noninvasively depict primary motor or sensory areas as well as language centers in patients prior to brain tumor surgery (Atlas et al. 1996; Mueller et al. 1996; Maldjian et al. 1996), epilepsy surgery (Chapman et al. 1995), radiosurgery (Latchaw et al. 1995), treatment of pain (Kiriakopoulos et al. 1996), and endovascular therapy (Maldjian et al. 1996). Despite their circumscribed appearance on conventional MRI, some astrocytomas are highly infiltrative. This may explain how a function can be partially (or, at the beginning, entirely) preserved. Identification of residual function is of great importance to the neurosurgeon as it permits maximizing tumor resection whilst minimizing post-operative morbidity. The degree of infiltration of the tumor is likely to influence the surrounding functional tissue. The pattern of activation seems to match the spatial classification of brain tumors according to their degree of infiltration (Kleihues et al. 1993). In type I circumscribed tumors, the cerebral activation is displaced by the tumor (Fig. 5). In type II or III infiltrating tumors, the activation is displaced and scattered. In type IV diffusely infiltrating tumors, the activation is fully scattered (Fig. 6). In a study involving seven patients with gliomas, Atlas et al. (1996) showed that functional cortex within or adjacent to tumor margins may correspond to partial preservation of clinical function and suggested that the activation could be quantified. Yousry et al. (1995) found a broader and more diffuse activated motor area in four patients with brain tumors compared to healthy volunteers. In similar studies involving intraoperative cortical mapping in 14 and 28 patients, respectively, Ojemann et al. (1996) and Skirboll et al. (1996) observed that the brain tissue surrounding an infiltrating tumor remains functional, precluding safe tumor resection.

Functional MRI has been repeated reproducibly in selected patients with congenital lesions such as arteriovenous malformation (AVM) or slowly growing brain tumors to study cortical reorganization phenomena. Ipsilateral or supplementory motor area activations seen in some of the slowly growing brain tumors could be related to such phenomena. Maldjian et al. (1996) investigated six patients with AVM and identified some unexpected functional areas, which could be attributed to brain function plasticity. The ability of fMRI to detect phenomena of cortical reorganization opens new prospects in the study of

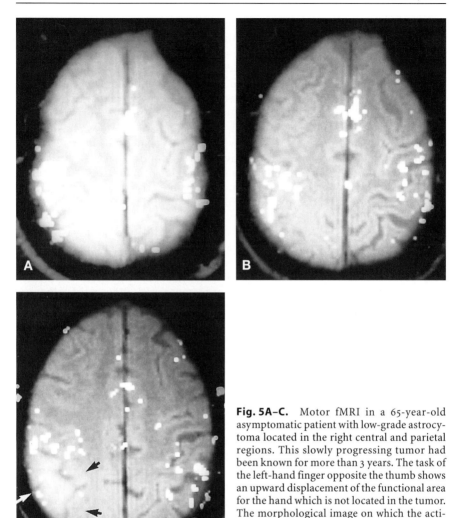

Fig. 5A–C. Motor fMRI in a 65-year-old asymptomatic patient with low-grade astrocytoma located in the right central and parietal regions. This slowly progressing tumor had been known for more than 3 years. The task of the left-hand finger opposite the thumb shows an upward displacement of the functional area for the hand which is not located in the tumor. The morphological image on which the activated pixels are superimposed allows visualization of the tumor (*arrows*), reflecting a slight hyperintensity and mass effect on the sulci

AVM or slowly growing lesions. It may even become possible to evaluate the recovery of motor function following tumor resection.

2.1.4.2 fMRI in Multiple Sclerosis (MS)

Structural imaging of demyelinating lesions with MRI in MS has provided new insights into the underlying pathophysiological mechanisms. MRI has become an invaluable tool for the clinical and therapeutic research in this field. However, high signal patches on T_2-weighted images indicate chemical modifica-

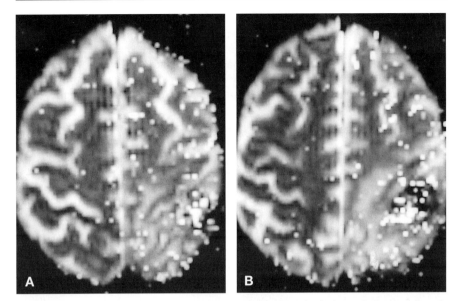

Fig. 6A, B. Motor fMRI in a 68-year-old patient with glioblastoma discovered after an acute episode related to a tumoral bleed. The task of the right-hand finger opposite the thumb produces an activation involving the tumoral bed, particularly at its posterior ridge. This 1.5-T FID-EPI image (effective TE 51 ms) was acquired with high resolution (field of view of 220 × 220 mm combined with a 96 × 128 matrix)

tion of the normal white matter without yielding any information regarding the activity of the lesion or its functional effects. The lack of correlation between high signal intensity and the clinical presentation of MS was one of the striking findings in the first reported studies (McFarland et al. 1992; Thompson et al. 1992). Moreover, demyelination has complex physiological properties: conduction block, decrease of conduction velocities, desynchronization of the bursts of action potentials, and ephaptic transmission. In MS the anatomo-clinical correlations are poor and many symptoms such as fatigue or neuropsychological disturbances are not clearly explained by the structural changes identified at morphological imaging (Rao et al. 1989). The development of the functional imaging techniques promise to help clarify the dynamic process which leads to the reversibility of symptoms and repair of brain damage.

Less attention has been paid to functional imaging of MS than to that of other diseases such as vascular, epileptic, or tumoral disorders. There are a few reports on the variations of distribution of regional cerebral blood flow induced by the demyelinating lesions and their correlations with neuropsychological symptoms. However, fMRI offers the opportunity of shedding light on the remote effects of demyelination. In conjunction with other MRI techniques, including spectroscopy, magnetization transfer, and diffusion imaging, early differentiation between irreversible lesions with axonal loss and reversible edematous or purely demyelinating lesions may become possible. Figure 7 presents some preliminary examples of functional images obtained by motor activation in MS patients which suggest that fMRI might anticipate the recovery of a motor deficit. In MS patients unable to move, no activation is visible.With partial motor weakness, patients activate larger motor areas than normal in both hemispheres: primary motor cortex bilaterally, contralateral premotor cortex, supplementary motor area, and some areas in the associa-

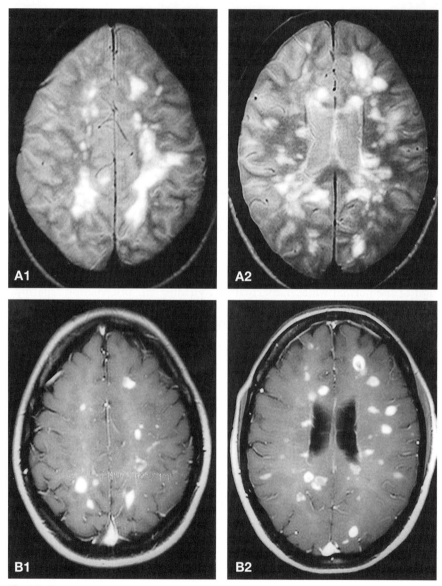

Fig. 7A–G

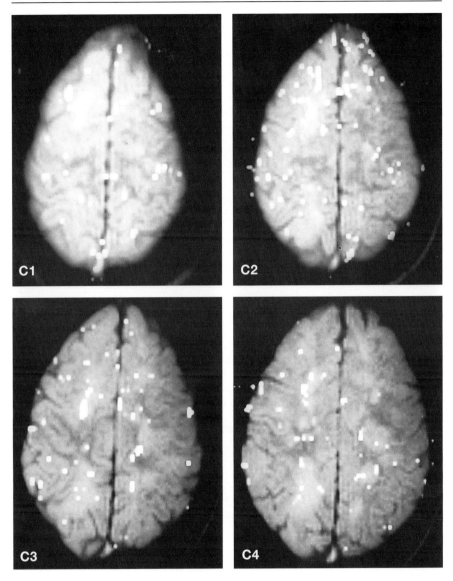

Fig. 7A–G. Motor fMRI in a patient with MS, illustrating cortical activity dependence upon axonal output capability. A 25-year-old woman with severe relapsing-remitting MS since 1989 had an exacerbation, with six relapses within 1 year. She entered the study during a relapse with gait disturbance, bilateral upper limb weakness (right hand totally impaired), right lower limb weakness, and ataxia of limbs (Expanded Disability Status Scale 4). T2-weighted images reveal a large lesion load (**A**) and extensive gadolinium enhancement (**B**). On fMRI no structured activation is observed associated with the immobile right hand (**C**). Movement of the left hand (**D**) activates the primary motor cortex in both hemispheres, demonstrating the functional integrity of both primary motor areas. As the patient progressively recovers her right-hand function, fMRI shows a restored activation in the left motor cortex. On follow-up MRI 2 months later there is persistent

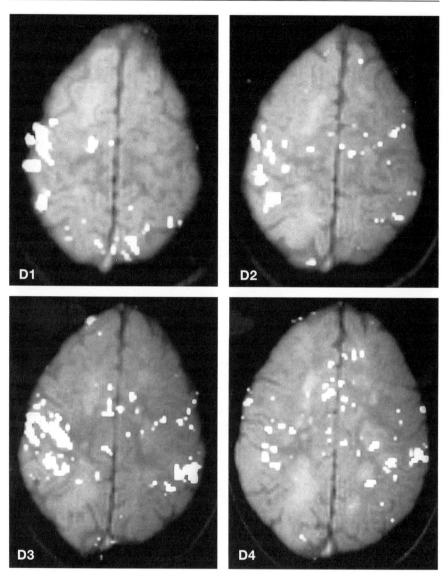

Fig. 7A–G

enhancement following injection of paramagnetic contrast (**E**). On fMRI the right hand now induces an activation with an enlarged and bilateral response (**F**). Activation associated with the left
hand remains unchanged (**G**)

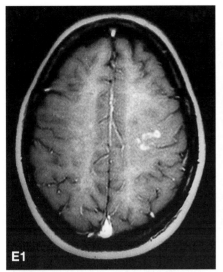 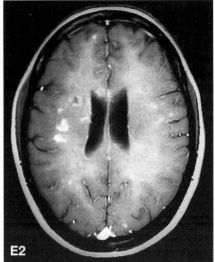

Fig. 7E

tive cortex. An acute inflammatory demyelinating lesion producing a conduction block recovery to paralyze the upper limb deactivates the primary motor cortex by an unclear mechanism. However, persistent functional capacity is proven by the increase in metabolic rate induced by the movements of the ipsilateral fingers. Functional MRI could thus emerge as one of the new tools allowing differentiation of the reversible functional deficits produced by pure demyelination from the definitive incapacitating symptoms secondary to axonal loss.

Several mechanisms have been implicated in the recovery of function in MS patients (Chollet and Weiller 1994). Among them, bilateral representation of function and extension of specialized areas are considered. In the case of a partial motor deficit, the activated surface area of the contralateral precentral gyrus is enlarged, as shown in patients following recovery from a vascular capsular lesion (Weiller et al. 1992). This adjacent recruitment may represent a cortical adaptation to pyramidal tract dysfunction. Serial follow-up of motor recovery after relapse in MS patients has shown the activated area to vary with the intensity of the functional deficit, suggesting that a dynamic component is inherent to the recovery process. At this time it remains unclear whether the recruitment of the ipsilateral sensorimotor cortex observed in the majority of patients with partial deficits actually corresponds to the recruitment of ipsilateral corticospinal pathways or represents a mere epiphenomenon related to artifactual mirror synkinetic movements.

MS is a complex disorder in which different destructive mechanisms impede the functional neurological sytems in a subtle way. Emerging treatments may modify the clinical course of these patients, and some new strategies for repairing the damage are under consideration (Compston 1994). Functional MRI

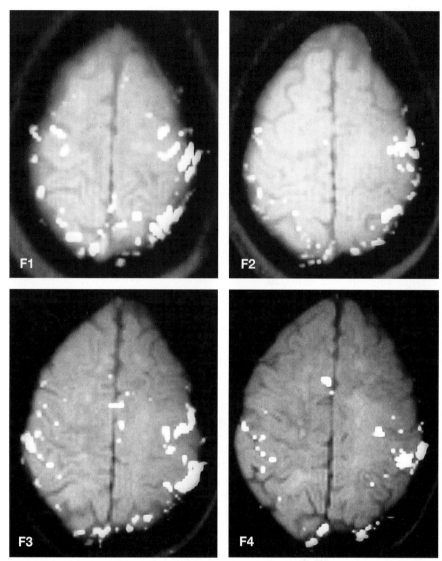

Fig. 7A–G

has the capacity to provide new clues which will allow further fine-tuning of
the different therapeutic approaches.

2.2   Perfusion Imaging of the Brain

The cerebral intravascular space makes up only 5% of the brain. Therefore,
extracting its contribution from the signal of the whole brain is difficult. Two

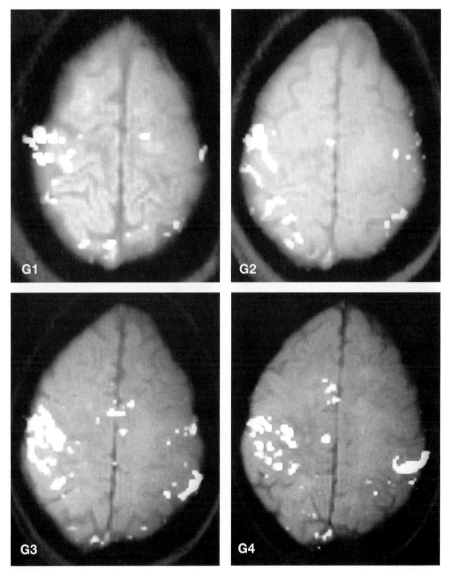

Fig. 7A–G

approaches allow amplification of the blood pool MR signal: perfusion tech-niques based on the differential velocities of water molecules (Le Bihan et al. 1988a) and use of contrast agents. The latter can either be imaged at stable blood concentrations [intravascular contrast agents] such as ultrasmall super-paramagnetic iron oxide particles, USPIO (Berry et al. 1996)], or rapidly imaged during their first passage, which is proportional to cerebral blood volume and cerebral blood flow (Villringer et al. 1988). Among fast imaging techniques employed to assess contrast perfusion, EPI techniques achieve the greatest temporal resolution, permitting the monitoring of the cerebrovascular transit of magnetic susceptibility-inducing contrast media (Fig. 8). The mechanism of such contrast media is completely different from the acceleration of T_1 relaxation exploited for morphologic purposes (blood-brain barrier assessment). Generally the same agents can serve both goals because of the high magnetic moment of gadolinium chelates. Reflecting considerable T_2 and T_2^* components, USPIO contrast also results in a considerable signal loss when used as a first-pass contrast agent in conjunction with EPI (Forsting et al. 1994). Magnetic susceptibility (T_2^*) contrast agents induce microscopic magnetic field inhomogeneities, resulting in a loss of signal intensity in perfused tissue. They allow dynamic comparison of the transit time in different territories (Fig. 8). Experimental evidence of perfusion defects is provided by the absence of a signal decrease during bolus passage. The hemodynamic consequence for the perfused but compressed part of an injured hemisphere is delayed and prolonged signal loss compared with the contralateral normal hemisphere (Maeda et al. 1993).

Relative quantification of cerebral blood volume is possible by integration of the area under the curve of signal evolution during the passage of the bolus (Röther et al. 1996). Perfusion deficits may be visualized within 1 h following vessel occlusion in stroke, i.e., before substantial pathological changes occur and prior to any reliable depiction of these deficits by standard proton MRI techniques. Standard T_2-weighted MRI without contrast enhancement typically fails to demonstrate any significant signal alterations before the onset of cerebral edema, which induces a relative signal increase approximately 4 h after vessel occlusion (Edelman et al. 1990; Warach et al. 1992a).

2.3   Diffusion-Weighted Imaging of the Brain

MR signal intensity is dependent among other factors on water motion, which intrinsically produces contrast. Diffusion-weighted imaging (DWI) exploits the range of velocities displacing water within the order of magnitude of the voxel size during an echo time. These velocities have been referred to as intravoxel incoherent motion, IVIM (Le Bihan et al. 1986). Imaging is sensitized to motion in the direction of additional gradients and characterized by 'b', the gradient factor. Such gradients diminish the signal intensity in proportion to Brownian diffusion in the direction in which they are applied. If one direction is sensitized, anisotropy of diffusion can be studied (Fig. 9). For a global evaluation, all three directions need to be sensitized. EPI is useful in this respect, as it permits exploration of several directions and several b factors in a small amount of time, thus limiting motion artifacts, to which these images are generally highly sensitive.

Most acute and/or evolutive lesions are associated with hyperintensity on DWI, reflecting a decrease of the apparent diffusion coefficient (ADC) of water in the injury (Le Bihan et al. 1988a) (Figs. 10, 11). This is related to disruption of energy metabolism and failure of the Na/K-ATPase sodium pump, lead-

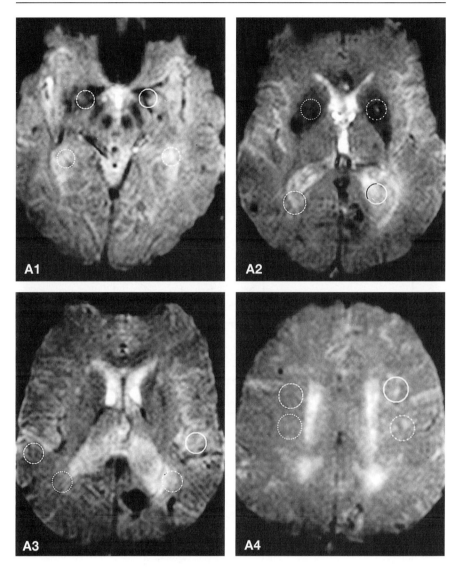

Fig. 8A,B.   Perfusion-weighted imaging in a 54-year-old man with left carotid stenosis. High-resolution FID-EPI images (effective TE 66 ms) acquired every 1 s for 20 s on four levels (field of view 220 × 220 mm in a matrix of 128 × 128) illustrate the circulation of an intravenously injected gadolinium chelate bolus. (B) Region of interest analysis of the time curve evolution of signal intensity. The decrease in signal is proportional to the tissue perfusion. Vascular and basal ganglia perfusion occurs early and symmetrical (**A1, A2** and matched curves on **B1, B2**). The left territory of the middle cerebral artery is revascularized by pial collaterals, and the corresponding curves (*arrows*) reveal a delay compared to the contralateral side (**B4**). There is a junctional infarction by hemodynamic insufficiency in the left temporo-parieto-occipital region (**A3**; *arrow*), and the contrast agent entry is very delayed (**B3**; *arrow*)

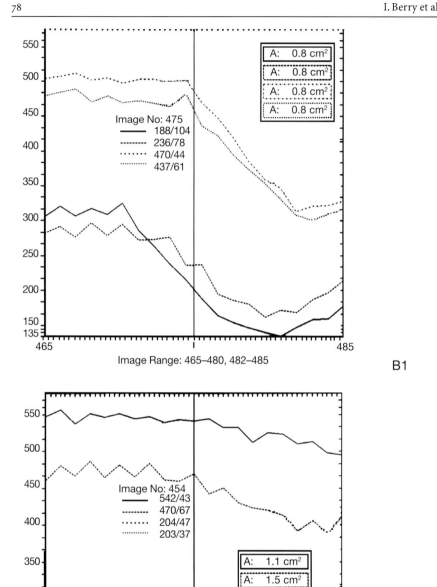

Image Range: 465–480, 482–485

B1

Image Range: 444–464

B2

Fig. 8B

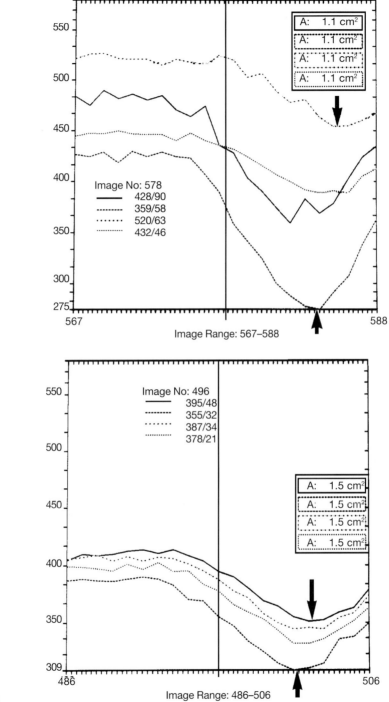

B3

Image No: 578
428/90
359/58
520/63
432/46

A: 1.1 cm²
A: 1.1 cm²
A: 1.1 cm²
A: 1.1 cm²

Image Range: 567–588

B4

Image No: 496
395/48
355/32
387/34
378/21

A: 1.5 cm²
A: 1.5 cm²
A: 1.5 cm²
A: 1.5 cm²

Image Range: 486–506

Fig. 8B

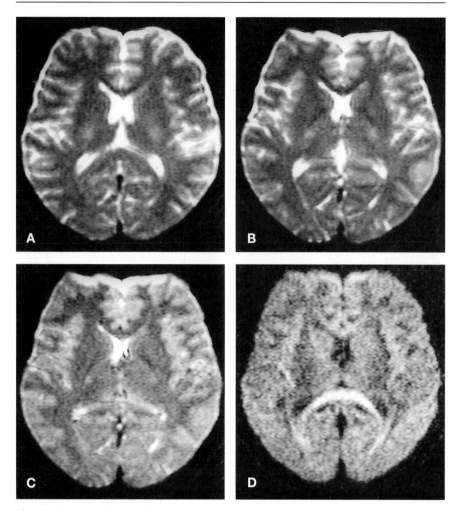

Fig. 9A–D. DWI of a normal volunteer demonstrating anisotropy of white matter fiber orientation. Five-millimeter-thick spin-echo EPI section (effective TE 123 ms), selected from five slices
acquired in 1.25 s, is acquired with a field of view of 210 × 210 mm in a matrix of 128 × 200. The
gradients of this 1.5 T Magnetom Vision (Siemens, Erlangen, Germany) can achieve a rise time of
300 ms to reach sinusoidally a maximum intensity of 25 mT/m. In this acquisition the signal is
sensitized to diffusion in the slice selection (cranio-caudal) direction by a gradient pulse of factor
b = 0 s/mm² (**A**), 30 s/mm² (**B**), 300 s/mm² (**C**), 1200 s/mm² (**D**). The highest b value (**D**) results in
a purely diffusion-weighted image, devoid of perfusion contribution to the signal. It reveals a
craniocaudal restriction in the path of water molecules in those structures oriented in the left-
right direction, including the genu and the splenium of the corpus callosum. There is also, to a
lesser extent, restriction of water motion in the craniocaudal direction in structures such as the
anterior limb of the internal capsule and the occipital white matter

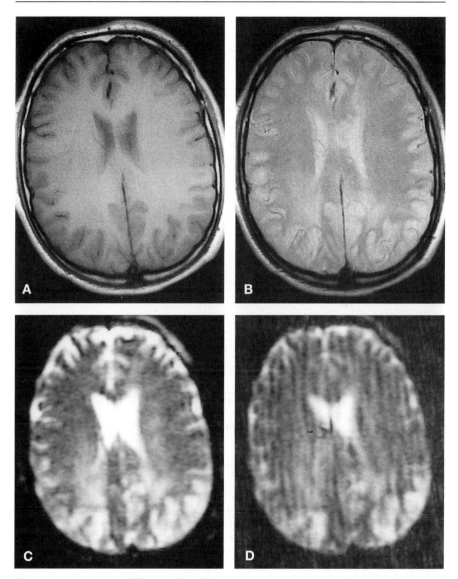

Fig. 10A–H. DWI early detection of anoxic lesions. A comatose 52-year-old man suffered a gaseous embolism following a diving accident 24 h prior to MRI. Neither T1-weighted imaging (**A**) nor a T2-weighted sequence (**B**) shows any abnormality. Diffusion-weighted MRI reveals cortical biocciptal and central gray matter anoxic lesions. The latter are better seen with the higher b values, reflecting more severely restricted diffusion of extracellular water due to cell swelling. Six-millimeter-thick spin-echo EPI section (effective TE 123 ms), collected in a series of 20 contiguous slices over 5.29 s with a field of view of 250×250 mm imaged in a 128×200 matrix. In this acquisition the signal is sensitized to diffusion in the three directions with successive gradient factor b values of 0 s/mm² (**C**), 600 s/mm² (**D**), 1370 s/mm² (**E**), 2500 s/mm² (**F**), 3087 s/mm² (**G**), and 4446 s/mm² (**H**)

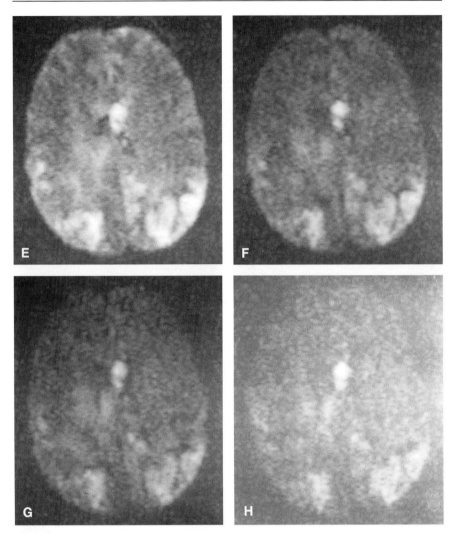

Fig. 10G–H

ing to loss of ion homeostasis and to early intracellular water accumulation, i.e., cytotoxic cell swelling (Moseley et al. 1990; Busza et al. 1992). Restriction of water diffusion is initially related to the decreased size of the extracellular space in the presence of cytotoxic edema. This decrease may be as high as 50%. A mechanism that has also been incriminated, but is probably observed only with the highest b values, reflects the larger amount of intracellular water. In the intracellular space diffusion is intrinsically more limited than in the extracellular space (Van Gelderen et al. 1994).

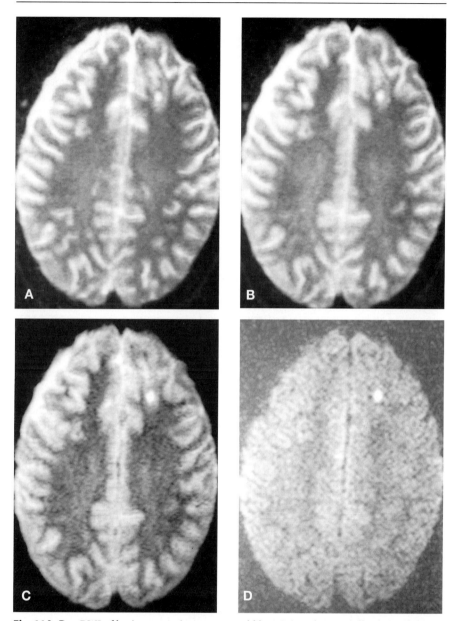

Fig. 11A–D.   DWI of brain trauma in an 11-year-old boy. Spin-echo EPI (effective TE 123 ms) with monodirectional sensitization of the signal to diffusion in the slice-select direction, with gradient pulse factors b = 0 s/mm² (**A**), 30 s/mm² (**B**), 300 s/mm² (**C**), and 1200 s/mm² (**D**). Five-millimeter slices selected from a series of 18 sections acquired in 4.38 s with a 128 × 200 matrix and a field of view of 210 × 210 mm. A punctate hemorrhagic lesion in the left frontal lobe shows a highly restricted diffusion coefficient. It is characterized by increased signal intensity compared to parenchyma and CSF on the highest b value image (**D**). The right frontal hygroma has elevated diffusion and presents with low signal intensity on this image

2.3.1 Application to the Early Diagnosis and Prognosis Determination of Stroke

Slowly, a consensus regarding the necessity of emergency MRI in stroke seems to be emerging. Early visualization of the lesion could improve the prognosis of this disease, but the choice of technique to best achieve this is still subject to controversy. In 1991, correlation of T1- and T2-weighted MRI and non-contrast-enhanced CT, performed within 3 h after stroke, showed no difference between the two methods (Mohr et al. 1995). CT is excellent for demonstration of early parenchyma modification and very reliable for depiction of hemorrhage, which is not as easy with MRI. In light of the new developments in MRI these findings and the conclusions drawn from them require reassessment.

Experimental stroke models have convincingly shown an early decrease in the apparent diffusion coefficient (ADC) in ischemic territories, prior to any signal alterations on T2-weighted images (Moseley et al. 1990a,b; Kucharczyk et al. 1991; Moonen et al. 1991; Berry et al. 1992). This is related to the characteristics of cytotoxic edema, which correlates well with the propagation of the infarction (Knight et al. 1994). A recent meta-analysis of experimental studies emphasized the sensitivity of DWI to acute stroke extension (Hoehn-Berlage 1995). Prognostic factors which have been identified include the volume of the lesion and the decrease in ADC. The latter has been shown to correlate with the local reduction in cerebral blood flow (Mancuso et al. 1995). ADC is decreased to a lesser extent in the penumbra than in the infarcted zone itself, and an ADC threshold of tissue viability will certainly be established.

Some clinical studies applying these concepts have already been undertaken. The first was reported by Warach et al. (1992a). In 4 of 32 patients, the infarct was seen only on DWI and initially not depicted on T2-weighted sequences. The same group subsequently reported whole-brain screening with multislice DWI-EPI in 3 s (Warach et al. 1995) (Fig. 12). The prognostic superiority of DWI over T2-weighted imaging was further confirmed in a series of 19 patients with extensive ischemic lesions. The ability to predict outcome was better with DWI (92% accuracy) than with T2-weighted imaging (33%) when performed within 6 h of the initial manifestation of stroke symptoms (Warach et al. 1996). Modeling of T2 and ADC evolution seems to be predictive of histological outcome of the tissue: cell recuperation or necrosis (Welch et al. 1995). Absence of signal changes on early DWI appears to be a good predictor of clinical recovery (Sorensen et al. 1996).

Dynamic susceptibility contrast MRI provides distinctive hemodynamic information about regions of ischemic penumbra, whereas on DWI it is difficult to distinguish normal regions from penumbra because of the small difference in ADC (Maeda et al. 1993). A combination of diffusion- and perfusion-sensitive MRI may thus be useful to assess regional alterations in ischemic brain injury following focal cerebrovascular occlusion (Quast et al. 1993; Fisher and Garcia 1996). The mismatch between the results of the two techniques is suspected to correspond to the penumbra. In many patients the initial lesion extension seen on DWI is smaller than the perfusion alteration as well as the changes seen later on T2 weighted images (Fisher and Garcia

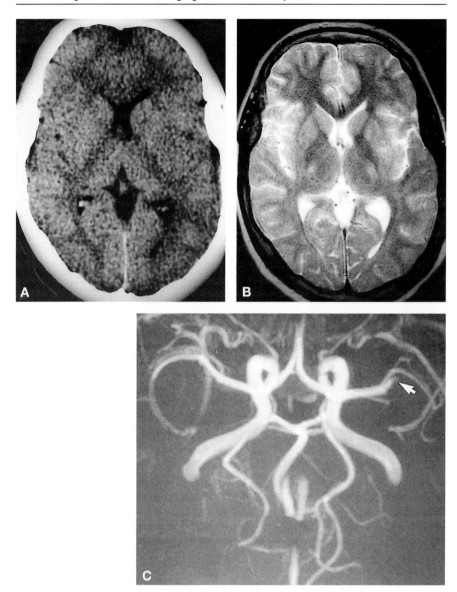

Fig. 12A–J. Hyperacute detection of stroke with DWI in a 24-year-old woman with sudden right hemiplegia who was 3 months pregnant. (**A**) Initial computed tomography performed 2 h after onset of clinical symptoms without contrast injection does not show any abnormality. (**B**) T2-weighted sequence performed with a fast spin-echo technique (TR 3800 ms, TE 17 ms, slice thickness 6 mm, field of view 188 × 250 mm, matrix 240 × 512, acquisition time 3 min 11 s) 5.5 h after onset of clinical symptoms is also within normal limits. (**C**) Early MR angiography confirms the occlusion of the left middle cerebral artery at the level of the bifurcation (*arrow*). (**D**) Diffusion-weighted spin-echo EPI (effective TE 123 ms, slice thickness 6 mm, field of view 250 × 250 mm, matrix 128 × 200, acquisition time 5.29 s for 20 slices) sensitized in the three directions by gradients of factor b = 0 s/mm² (**D1**), 1370 s/mm² (**D2**), 2500 s/mm² (**D3**), and 3087 s/mm² (**D4**) reveals

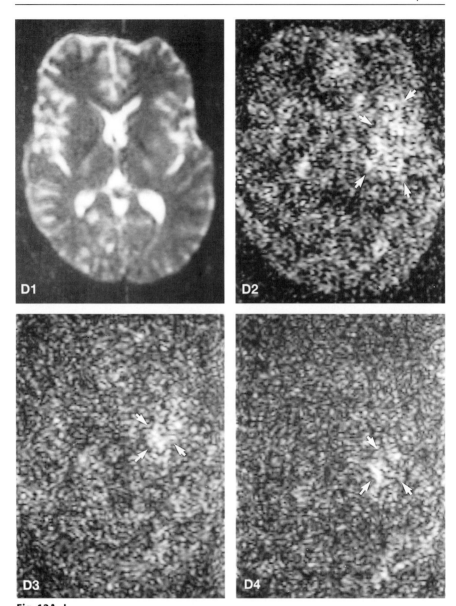

Fig. 12A–J

increased signal intensity in the left putamen (*arrows*) related to a local restriction of the diffusion of water molecules consistent with a cytotoxic edema build-up due to dysfunction of the membrane sodium pumps. At 48 h the patient was clinically recovered, without any functional deficit. At this time computed tomography (**E**) shows a left posterior putaminal hypodensity (*arrows*). T2-weighted MR image (**F**) shows an edematous lesion in the territory found to be abnormal on the early diffusion image. Revascularization of the left middle cerebral artery branches are confirmed on repeat MR angiography (**G**). Spin-echo EPI (**H**, b = 0 s/mm²; **I**, 2500 s/mm²) shows the

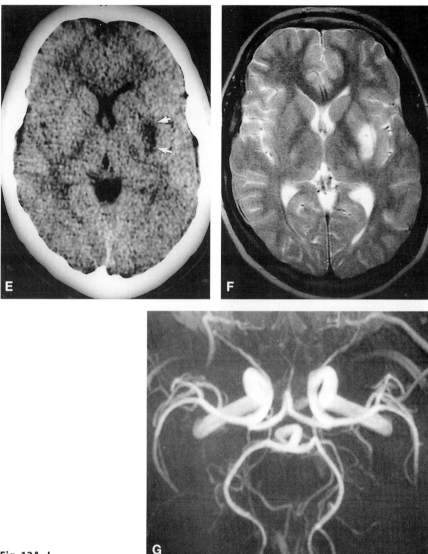

Fig. 12A–J

extent of the area of restricted diffusion with increased signal intensity. The respective roles of the T2 prolongation and the diffusion restriction in this lesion are separated by the calculation of the apparent diffusion coefficient image (**J**) with $ADC = Log(S_o/S_1)/(b_1-b_o)$ in mm²/s (S_o and S_1 are the signal intensities with the diffusion gradients of, respectively, b_o and b_1). Decreased ADC in the lesion indicates restricted diffusion (*arrows*). In this pregnant patient no iodine or gadolinium chelate could be injected to assess the blood-brain barrier and demonstrate the amount of vasogenic edema, which was minimal in the T2 prolongation of this asymptomatic lesion

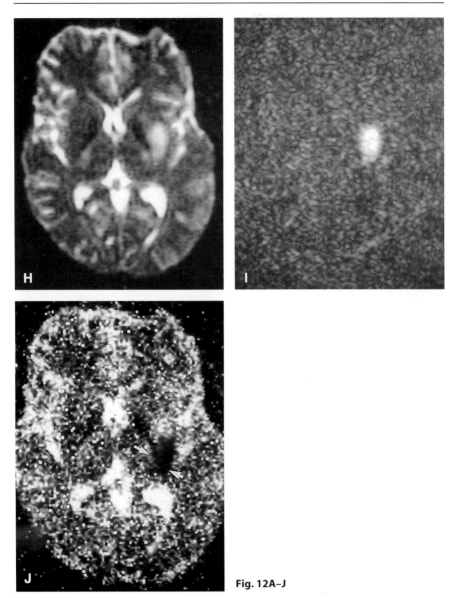

Fig. 12A–J

1996). A region of hypoperfusion larger than the region of diffusion abnormality may be predictive of ischemic lesion enlargement (Baird et al. 1997). A decreased diffusion coefficient during the hyperacute phase of experimental ischemia may, on the other hand, be present in regions where perfusion is still preserved. The diffusion abnormality is probably still reversible at this stage (Quast et al. 1993).

2.3.2   Application to MS

Multiple sclerosis disrupts the structure of the brain tissue by a combination of demyelination and axonal loss. Studies of pathology specimens showed a wide diversity in lesion presentation (Newcombe et al. 1991; Barnes et al. 1991; Lucchinetti et al. 1996). The extracellular space can be enlarged by myelin loss or restricted by dense gliosis. Abnormal diffusion characteristics can thus be expected to characterize this disease. Reflecting the small lesion size and motion sensitivity of the spin-echo DWI technique, MS has to date been the subject of only few DWI studies. The first report was by Christiansen et al. (1992), who found higher ADC in MS plaques than in normal appearing white matter. They also found higher ADC values in acute compared to chronic plaques. This was interpreted as related to an increase in the extracellular space reflecting the occurrence of edema and demyelination. In a more recent study patients with benign MS (mild disability) and secondary progressive MS (marked disability) were studied using a DWI technique less prone to artifacts. DWI substantiated the hypothesis that patients with greater disability are more likely to have more destructive lesions (Horsfield et al. 1996). While lesions from both groups showed an elevated diffusion coefficient, no statistically significant differences were found between the two groups. Normal appearing white matter in these patients had a higher ADC than that found in normal subjects, suggesting the presence of microscopic lesions below the spatial resolution of the images (Figs. 13, 14).

2.4   Magnetization Transfer Imaging

Recently, magnetization transfer (MT)-weighted MRI was recognized as a potentially important tool to characterize myelin of the brain. Indeed, MT contrast (MTC) MRI reflects the macromolecular content of tissue through the exchange of water molecules. This exchange takes place between a pool of water molecules bound to the macromolecules and mobile water contained within the interstitium. In standard imaging experiments, protons of bound water contribute little to the MR signal because of their short T2. Mobile protons on the other hand contribute the most (Wolff and Balaban 1989, 1994; Wolff et al. 1991; Ordidge et al. 1991). In the case of cerebral white matter, water molecules bound to myelin have a minimal direct influence on the signal (Koenig et al. 1990). Reflecting the high organization of macromolecular structure, MT from myelin protons is pronounced, producing high magnetization transfer ratios (MTR) (Fralix et al. 1991; Koenig 1991; Kucharczyk et al. 1994) (Fig. 15). The MTR of the myelin depends on age, and databases for reference values are currently being established (Silver et al. 1997).

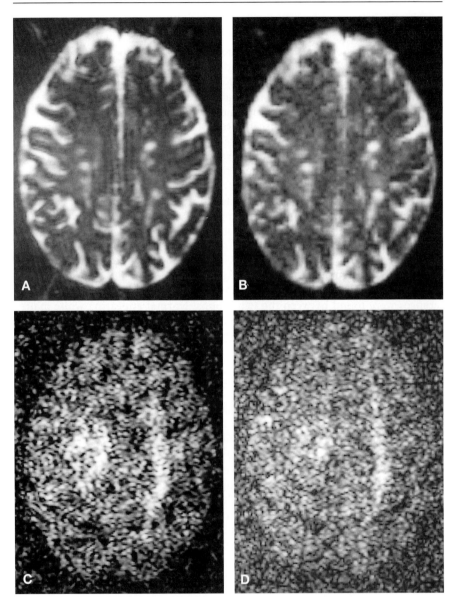

Fig. 13A–D. DWI of MS in a 47-year-old patient with the relapsing-remitting form of disease. Diffusion-weighted spin-echo EPI (effective TE 123 ms, slice thickness 5 mm, field of view 250 × 250 mm, matrix 128 × 200, acquisition time 8.66 s for 28 slices) sensitized in the three directions by gradients of factor b = 0 s/mm² (**A**), 600 s/mm² (**B**), 2500 s/mm² (**C**), and 3087 s/mm² (**D**). MS plaques are seen to be scattered in the white matter of the centrum semiovale on the T2-weighted image (**A**). Diffusely abnormal signal intensity in the white matter, including normal appearing parts, seen on the images with the highest b values is related to changes of the diffusion of water molecules (**C**, **D**)

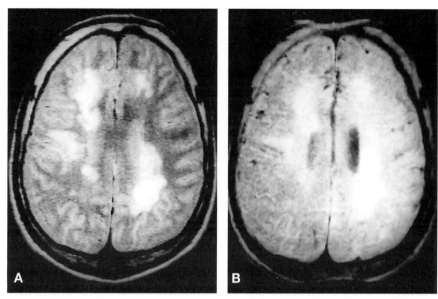

Fig. 14A, B. DWI of MS in a 24-year-old man. **A** Fast spin-echo TR 3800, TE 16 ms, rectangular field of view (224 × 256 mm) and matrix (224 × 256), acquisition time 2.56 min. **B** Steady-state gradient-echo sequence (TR 21.6 ms, TE 5 ms) sensitized anteroposteriorly in the phase-encoding direction by a gradient whose b factor is 800 s/mm². This 5-mm-thick slice is acquired in 3.2 s with a field of view of 180 × 240 mm and a matrix of 144 × 256. This diffusion-weighted technique shows diffusely abnormal signal intensity in the plaques as well as in the normal appearing white matter

2.4.1 Echo-Planar Generation of MT Maps

MT-sensitized techniques such as spin echo or gradient echo have so far allowed calculation of the MTR. However, these techniques usually do not permit clear visualization of inhomogeneities of MTR on multislice imaging. Indeed, the signal to noise ratio is usually too limited with conventional spin-echo or gradient-echo data collection to accurately reflect subtle differences on MTR maps. Nevertheless, this parameter seems useful in studying the extent and pattern of focal lesions. EPI with the addition of an MT pulse (MT-EPI) provides high temporal resolution, limiting motion artifacts which characterize most conventional acquisition schemes. MT-EPI maps of the entire brain can be generated with adequate signal-to-noise in less than 2 min (Ranjeva et al. 1996) (Fig. 16).

2.4.2 Evaluation of Demyelination in MS

Due to a larger pool of mobile water molecules, lesions of the white matter, e.g., MS, generally exhibit prolongation of the T2 relaxation time. The origin

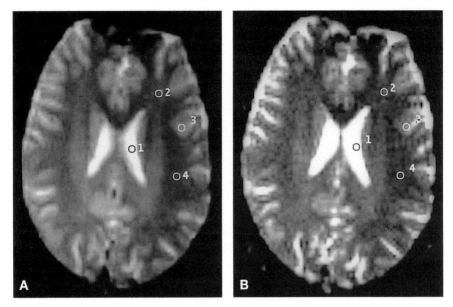

Fig. 15A, B. MT-weighted EPI in a normal volunteer. The MT preparation is achieved by a 25-MT pulse train (1.2 kHz off-water resonance, BW 500 Hz FWHM, duration 7620 ms, flip angle 55°, interpulse delay 5.5 ms) placed prior to an EPI-FID sequence (effective TE 66 ms, matrix 128 × 128, field of view 280 × 280 mm). MT-weighted imaging is obtained with two series of ten averaged measurements, one without (**A**) and the other with (**B**) MT preparation. Intermeasurement delay is 5 s to minimize saturation effects, each measurement lasting 1.55 s without MT preparation and 4.83 s with MT preparation for ten levels of 5-mm-thick slices. The MTR (%) is calculated as follows: $100 \ (S_o - S_{sat})/S_o$, where S_o is signal intensity acquired without MT saturation and S_{sat} is signal intensity obtained with MT saturation. Regions of interest are located (*1*) in the cerebrospinal fluid, collected as a control of a pool of fully free water without saturation transfer, and (*2–4*) in the white matter, which is expected to have the highest saturation transfer capabilities with its large pool of bound water adsorbed on the myelin sheaths. MTR: *1*, 6.6%; *2*, 60.4%; *3*, 58.5%; *4*, 59.0%

of the excess molecules lies in the presence of edema, and/or demyelination resulting in an increased interstitial space. Although differentiation between these two possible causes has functional implications, it is not possible using conventional T2-weighted imaging. Interestingly, MTR seems to have the potential to make this distinction, because demyelination, a more destructive process than edema, has been shown to lower MTR more than edema does (Dousset et al. 1992, 1995; Grossman 1994; Hiele et al. 1995; Tomiak et al. 1994; Campi et al. 1996) (Fig. 17). This explains why MTR has already been shown to correlate better with the Expanded Disability Status Scale (reflecting handicap) than do conventional T2-weighted sequences (Gass et al. 1994).

The fixation of the extracellular contrast agent gadolinium in MS lesions is related to vasogenic edema and not to demyelination. Hypothetically, the inflammatory lesions (edema) still have an organized macromolecular structure; the blood-brain barrier may or may not remain intact. At this stage the nature

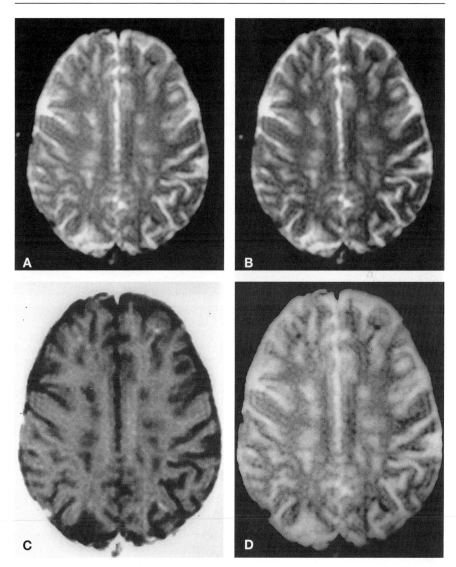

Fig. 16A–D. EPI-MT weighted sequence in a patient with MS. The MT preparation, acquired as in Figure 15, is integrated into an EPI-FID sequence (effective TE 29 ms, matrix 128 × 128, field of view 240 × 240 mm, 0.68 and 2.29 s acquisition times for five levels of 5-mm-thick slices). The acquisitions consist of two series of ten measurements each. One series is collected without and the other with MT preparation. Intermeasurement delay is 5 s to minimize saturation effects. In order to increase the signal-to-noise ratio and MT map accuracy, average images are calculated with the ten measurements performed for the two series: without (**A**) and with (**B**) MT preparation. Afterwards the MT maps (**C**) are reconstructed pixel by pixel according to MTR values (see Fig. 15). Display of the gray scale can be inverted (**D**) for better demonstration of lesion inhomogeneity. MS plaques contain demyelination, a destructive process which lowers the MTR, producing low signal intensity on MT maps (**C**)

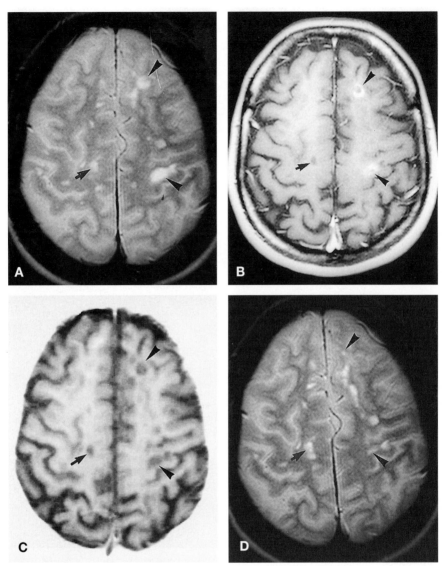

Fig. 17A–F. MT-weighted EPI sequence in a patient with MS. Selected MR images acquired 6 months apart show that acute lesions remain more structured than chronic ones with a large gliotic component. (**A, D**) T2-weighted images. (**B, E**) T1-weighted images following intravenous administration of paramagnetic contrast. (**C, F**) MT maps, same technique as Figure 16. On initial MRI some lesions indicate chronic demyelination with gliosis (*arrows*). They are hyperintense on T2-weighted images, hypointense on T1-weighted images, and have a very low MTR (very low signal intensity on **C**). Other lesions are acute (new lesion in the left central gyrus, reactivated lesion in the left anterior frontal white matter; *arrowheads*). They enhance following contrast injection and appear slighly dark on the MT map (moderately decreased MTR mostly due to an increase in the free water content unrelated to a demyelination process). The left frontal reactivated lesion (with rim enhancement) is inhomogeneous because it comprises both edema and

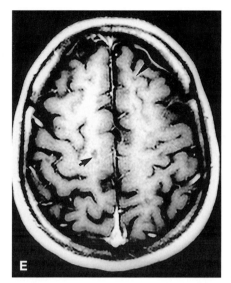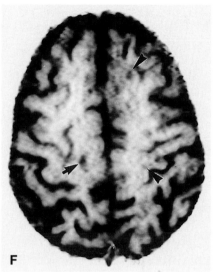

demyelination, which combine their mechanisms to largely decrease the MTR. Six months later the left anterior frontal lesion is gliotic (*arrowhead*) with less extensive hyperintensity on the T2-weighted image (**D**), marked hypointensity on the T1-weighted image (**E**), and very low MTR (**F**). The plaque of the left central gyrus presents limited demyelination with a quasi-recovered appearance on the MTR map (**F**; *arrowhead*)

of the myelin structure is characterized by a large MTR, almost equivalent to that of normal tissue (42% vs 47% for normal white matter) (Mehta et al. 1996). In these conditions, the MT processes (the chemical exchange and the nuclear Overhauser effect, NOE) constitute a major influence on the relaxation mechanisms. They induce a large decrease in the MR signal under MT saturation. In contrast, older gliotic lesions contain less organized structures with an elevated free water content in a large interstitial compartment and destruction of the myelin sheath. As a consequence, their MTR is very low (10–15%). This small contribution of the MT effect to the relaxation process is mainly due to a lack of bound protons, which prevents the chemical exchange of the magnetization between the different pools and cancels out the NOE because of the larger distance between protons.

Comparisons of gadolinium-enhancement in MS lesions and MTR values on respective MT maps reveal a coherent correlation between acute and chronic lesions. Older lesions present with a low MTR related to demyelination. Newly formed lesions have moderately low MTR reflecting the presence of edema, which increases the size of the free water compartment. Reactivated lesions presenting with rim enhancement have a very low MTR due to the combined effects of edema and demyelination.

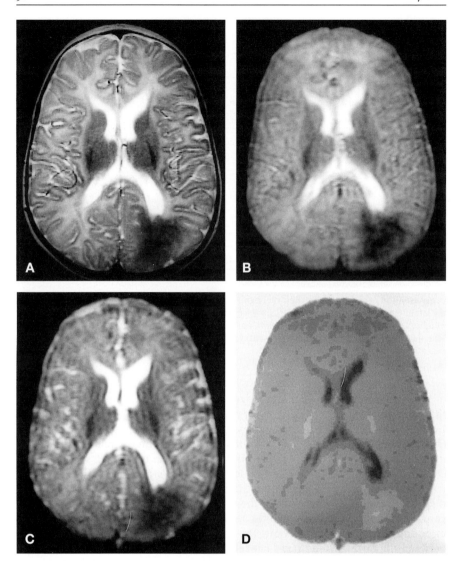

Fig. 18A–D. MT imaging of Bourneville tuberous sclerosis in a 5-month-old boy. **A** T2-weighted fast spin-echo image (TR 4000 ms, TE 120 ms, 5-mm-thick slice, field of view 150 × 200 mm, matrix 180 × 256, acquisition time 1.40 min). MT-weighted EPI is acquired as in Fig. 16. Measurement duration for 15 slices is 1.96 s without MT preparation and 4.83 s with MT preparation. **B** EPI without MT preparation. **C** MT-prepared EPI. **D** MTR map. Myelination of white matter decreases signal intensity on T2-weighted image and increases MTR. This is observed in the posterior limb of the internal capsule at this age. Left temporo-occipital tuber: a structured lesion presents with low signal intensity on T2-weighted imaging and a high MTR

2.4.3 Brain Malformations

MT has been shown to reveal more tubers and white matter lesions than conventional sequences in patients with Bourneville tuberous sclerosis (Zimmerman and Girard 1995). Subependymal nodules and cortical tubers may show low MTR, resembling values of gray matter. This is related to the associated heterotopia of gray matter. In developing brain, the conjunction of the myelination process and the presence of tubers produce foci of higher MTR (Fig. 18).

References

Atlas SW, Howard RS II, Maldjian J et al (1996) Functional magnetic resonance imaging of regional brain activity in patients with intracerebral gliomas: findings and implications for clinical management. Neurosurgery 38:329–338

Baird AE, Benfield A, Schlaug G et al (1997) Enlargement of human cerebral ischemic lesion volumes measured by diffusion-weighted magnetic resonance imaging. Ann Neurol 41:581–589

Baker PN, Johnson IR, Gowland PA et al (1995) Measurement of fetal liver, brain and placental volumes with echo-planar magnetic resonance imaging. Br J Obstet Gynaecol 102:35–39

Bandettini PA, Wong EC, Hinks RS, Tikofsky RS, Hyde JS (1992) Time course EPI of human brain function during task activation. Magn Reson Med 25:390–397

Barnes D, Munro PMG, Youl BD, Prineas JW, McDonald WI (1991) The longstanding MS lesion. Brain 114:1271–1280

Belliveau JW, Rosen BR, Kantor HL et al (1990) Functional cerebral imaging by susceptibility-contrast NMR. Magn Reson Med 14:538–546

Belliveau JW, Kennedy DN, McKinstry RC et al (1991) Functional mapping of the human visual cortex by magnetic resonance imaging. Science 254:716–719

Berry I, Gigaud M, Manelfe C (1992) Experimental focal cerebral ischemia assessed with IVIM*-MRI in the acute phase at 0.5 tesla. Neuroradiology 34:135–140

Berry I, D•monet J-F, Warach S et al (1995) Activation of association auditory cortex demonstrated with functional MRI. Neuroimage 2:215–219

Berry I, Benderbous S, Ranjeva JP, Gracia-Meavilla D, Manelfe C, Le Bihan D (1996) Contribution of USPIO used as blood-pool contrast agent: detection of cerebral blood volume changes during apnea in rabbit. Magn Reson Med 36:415–419

Binder JR, Rao SM, Hammeke TA et al (1993) Temporel characteristics of functional magnetic resonance signal change in lateral frontal and auditory cortex. Society of Magnetic Resonance in Medicine, 12th Annual Scientific meeting, New York

Binder JR, Rao SM, Hammeke TA et al (1994) Functional magnetic resonance imaging of human auditory cortex. Ann Neurol 35:662–672

Boecker H, Kleinschmidt A, Weindl A, Conrad B, Hšnicke W, Frahm J (1994) Dysfunctional activation of subcortical nuclei in palatal myoclonus detected by high-resolution MRI. NMR Biomed 7:327–329

Bucher SF, Seelos KC, Stehling M, Oertel WH, Paulus W, Reiser M (1995) High resolution activation mapping of basal ganglia with functional magnetic resonance imaging. Neurology 45:180–182

Busza A, Allen K, King M et al (1992) Diffusion-weighted imaging studies of cerebral ischemia in gerbils: potential relevance to energy failure. Stroke 23:1602–1612

Campi A, Filippi M, Comi G, Scotti G, Gerevini S, Dousset V (1996) Magnetisation transfer ratios of contrast-enhancing and nonenhancing lesions in multiple sclerosis. Neuroradiology 38:115–119

Chapman PM, Buchbinder BR, Cosgrove GR, Jiang MF (1995) Functional magnetic resonance imaging for cortical mapping in pediatric neurosurgery. Pediatr Neurosurg 23:122–126

Chollet F, Weiller C (1994) Imaging recovery of function following brain injury. Curr Opin Neurobiol 4:226–230

Christiansen P, Gideon P, Thomsen C, Stubgaard M, Henriksen O, Larsson HBW (1992) Increased water self-diffusion in chronic plaques and in apparently normal white matter in patients with multiple sclerosis. Acta Neurol Scand 87:195-199

Cohen JD, Forman SD, Braver TS, Casey BJ, Servan-Schreiber D, Noll DC (1994) Activation of the prefrontal cortex in a nonspatial working memory task with functional MRI. Hum Brain Mapp 1:293-304

Cohen MS, Bookheimer SY (1994) Localization of brain function using magnetic resonance imaging. Trends Neurosci 17:268-277

Colletti P-M, Sylvestre P-B (1994) Magnetic resonance imaging in pregnancy. Magn Reson Imaging Clin North Am 2:291-307

Compston A (1994) Brain repair: an overview. J Neurol 241:S1-S4

Connely A, Jackson GD, Frackowiak RSJ, Belliveau JW, Vargha-Khadem F, Gadian DG (1993) Functional mapping of activated human primary cortex with a clinical MR imaging system. Radiology 188:125-130

Constable R, McCarthy G, Allison T, Anderson AW, Gore JC (1993) Functional brain imaging at 1.5 T using conventional gradient echo MR imaging techniques. Magn Reson Imaging 11:451-459

D'Ercole C, Girard N, Boublin, Potier A et al (1993) Prenatal diagnosis of fetal cerebral abnormalities by ultrasonography and magnetic resonance imaging. Eur J Obstet Gynecol Reprod Biol 50:177-184

Damasio AR (1994) Descartes' error. Emotion, reason and the human brain. Grosset/Putnam, New York

de Coene B, Hajnal JV, Gatehouse P et al (1992) MR of the brain using fluid-attenuated inversion recovery (FLAIR) pulse sequences. AJNR 13:1555-1564

Deiber M-P, Passingham RE, Colebatch JG, Friston KJ, Nixon PD, Frackowiak RSJ (1991) Cortical areas and the selection of movement: a study with positron emission tomography. Exp Brain Res 84:393-402

Demonet JF, Chollet F, Ramsay S et al (1992) The anatomy of phonological and semantic processing in normal subjects. Brain 115:1753-1768

Dousset V, Grossman RI, Ramer KN et al (1992) Experimental allergic encephalomyelitis and multiple sclerosis: lesion characterization with magnetization transfer imaging. Radiology 182:483-491

Dousset V, Brochet B, Vital A et al (1995) Lysolecithin-induced demyelination in primates: preliminary in vivo study with MR and magnetization transfer. Am J Neuroradiol 16:225-231

Edelman RR, Mattle HP, Atkinson DJ et al (1990) Cerebral blood flow: assessment with dynamic contrast-enhanced T2* weighted MR imaging at 1.5T. Radiology 176:211-220

Engel SA, Rumelhart DE, Wandell BA et al (1994) fMRI of human visual cortex. Nature 369:525

Fisher M, Garcia JH (1996) Evolving stroke and the ischemic penumbra. Neurology 47:884-888

Forsting M, Reith W, Dšfler A et al (1994) MRI in acute cerebral ischemia: perfusion imaging with superparamagnetic iron oxide in a rat model. Neuroradiology 36:23-26

Frahm J, Merboldt KD, HŠnicke W (1993) Functional MRI of human brain activation at high spatial resolution. Magn Reson Med 29:139-144

Fralix TA, Ceckler TL, Wolff SD, Simon SA, Balaban RS (1991) Lipid bilayer and water proton magnetization transfer: effect of cholesterol. Magn Reson Med 18:214-223

Friston KJ, Holmes AP, Worsley KJ, Poline JB, Frith CD, Frackowiak RSJ (1995) Statistical parametric maps in functional imaging: a general approach. Hum Brain Mapp 2:189-210

Garden AS, Griffiths RD, Weindling AM, Martin PA (1991) Fast-scan magnetic resonance imaging in fetal visualization. Am J Obstet Gynecol 164:1190-1196

Gass A, Barker GJ, Kidd D et al (1994) Correlation of magnetization transfer ratio with clinical disability in multiple sclerosis. Ann Neurol 36:62-67

Girard N, Raybaud C (1992) In vivo MRI of foetal brain cellular migration. J Comput Assist Tomogr 16:265-267

Girard N, Raybaud C, Poncet M (1995) In vivo MR study of brain maturation in normal fetuses. AJNR 16:407-413

Grossman RI (1994) Magnetization transfer in multiple sclerosis. Ann Neurol 36:S97-S99

Guyer R, Hochschuler S, Spivey M, Ohnmeiss D, Castelman C (1992) The use of dynamic magnetic resonance imaging to identify cervical spine disc herniation and cord compression. A case report. Spine 17:596-597

Hammeke TA, Yetkin FZ, Mueller WM, Morris GL, Haughton VM, Rao SM, Binder JR (1994) Functional magnetic resonance imaging of somatosensory stimulation. Neurosurgery 35:677-681

Hiele JF, Grossman RI, Ramer KN, Gonzalez-Scarano F, Cohen JA (1995) Magnetization transfer effects in MR-detected multiple sclerosis lesions: comparison with gadolinium-enhanced spin-echo images and nonehanced T1-weighted images. Am J Neuroradiol 16:69-77

Hoehn-Berlage M (1995) Diffusion-weighted NMR imaging: applications to experimental focal cerebral ischemia. NMR Biomed 8:345–358

Horsfield MA, Lai M, Webb SL et al (1996) Apparent diffusion coefficients in benign and secondary progressive multiple sclerosis by nuclear magnetic resonance. Magn Reson Med 36:393–400

Jack CR, Thompson M, Butts RK et al (1994) Sensory motor cortex: correlation of presurgical mapping with functional MR imaging and invasive cortical mapping. Radiology 190:85–92

Kanal E (1994) Pregnancy and the safety of magnetic resonance imaging. Magn Reson Imaging Clin North Am 2:309–317

Kim S-G, Ugurbil K, Strick PL (1994) Activation of a cerebellar output nucleus during cognitive processing. Science 265:949–951

Kiriakopoulos ET, Wood ML, Mikulis DJ (1996) Functional magnetic resonance imaging and assessment of implanted neurostimulators. Neuroimage 4:S341

Kleihues P, Buerger PC, Scheithauer BW (1993) The new WHO classification of brain tumors. Brain Pathol 3:255–268

Kleinschmidt A, Merboldt K-D, HŠnicke W, Steinmetz H, Frahm J (1994) Correlational imaging of thalamocortical coupling in the primary visual pathway of the human brain. J Cereb Blood Flow Metab 14:952–957

Knight RA, Dereski MO, Helpern JA, Ordidge RJ, Chopp M (1994) Magnetic resonance imaging assessment of evolving focal cerebral ischemia. Comparison with histopathology in rats. Stroke 25:1252–1262

Koenig SH (1991) Cholesterol of myelin is the determinant of grey-white contrast in MRI of brain. Magn Reson Med 20:285–291

Koenig SH, Brown RD III, Spiller M, Lundbom N (1990) Relaxometry of brain: why white matter appears bright in MRI. Magn Reson Med 14:482–495

Koroshetz WJ, Gonzalez G (1997) Diffusion-weighted MRI: an ECG for "brain attack"? Ann Neurol 41:565–566

Kucharczyk J, Mintorovitch J, Asgari HS, Moseley M (1991) Diffusion/perfusion MR imaging of acute cerebral ischemia. Magn Reson Med 19:311–315

Kucharczyk W, Macdonald PM, Stanisz GJ, Henkelman RM (1994) Relaxivity and magnetization transfer of white matter lipids at MR imaging: importance of cerebrosides and pH. Radiology 192:521–529

Kwong KK, Belliveau JW, Chesler DA et al (1992) Dynamic magnetic resonance imaging of human brain activity during primary sensory stimulation. Proc Natl Acad Sci USA 89:5675–5679

Latchaw RE, Hu X, Ugurbil K, Hall WA, Madison MT, Heros RC (1995) Functional magnetic resonance imaging as a management tool for cerebral arteriovenous malformation. Neurosurgery 37:619–626

Le Bihan D, Breton E, Lallemand D, Grenier P, Cabanis E, Laval-Jeantet M (1986) MR imaging of intravoxel incoherent motions: application to diffusion and perfusion in neurologic disorders. Radiology 161:401–407

Le Bihan D, Breton E, Lallemand D, Aubin ML, Vignaud J, Laval-Jeantet M (1988a) Separation of diffusion and perfusion in intravoxel incoherent motion MR imaging. Radiology 168:497–505

Le Bihan D, Breton E, Lallemand D (1988b) MR imaging of intravoxel incoherent motions: application to diffusion and perfusion in neurologic disorders. Radiology 161:401–406

Lucchinetti CF, BrŸck W, Rodriguez M, Lassmann H (1996) Distinct patterns of multiple sclerosis pathology indicates heterogeneity in pathogenesis. Brain Pathol 6:259–274

Maeda M, Itoh S, Ide H et al (1993) Acute stroke in cats: comparison of dynamic susceptibility-contrast MR imaging with T2-and diffusion-weighted MR imaging. Radiology 189:227–232

Maldjian J, Atlas SW, Howard RS II et al (1996) Functional magnatic resonance imaging of regional brain activity in patients with intracerebral arteriovenous malformations before surgical or endovascular therapy. J Neurosurg 84:477–483

Mancuso A, Karibe H, Rooney WD et al (1995) Correlation of early reduction in the apparent diffusion coefficient of water with blood flow reduction during middle cerebral artery occlusion in rats. Magn Reson Med 34:368–377

McCarthy G, Blamire AM, Rothman DL, Gruetter R, Shulman RG (1993) Echo-planar magnetic resonance imaging studies of frontal cortex activation during word generation in humans. Proc Natl Acad Sci USA 90:4952–4956

McFarland HF, Frank JA, Albert PS et al (1992) Using gadolinium-enhanced magnetic resonance imaging lesions to monitor disease activity in multiple sclerosis. Ann Neurol 32:758–766

Mehta RC, Pike B, Enzmann DR (1996) Measure of magnetization transfer in multiple sclerosis demyeli-
    nating plaques, white matter ischemic lesions and edema. AJNR 17:1051-1055
Menon RS, Ogawa S, Tank DW, Ugurbil K (1993) 4 Tesla gradient recalled echo characteristics of photic
    stimulation-induced signal changes in the human primary visual cortex. Magn Reson Med 30:380-386
Mohr JP, Biller J, Hilal SK et al (1995) Magnetic resonance versus computed tomographic imaging in acute
    stroke. Stroke 26:807-812
Moonen CTW, Pekar J, De Vleeschouwer MHM, Van Gelderen P, Van Zijl PCM, Despres D (1991) Restricted
    and anisotropic displacement of water in healthy cat brain and in stroke studied by NMR diffusion
    imaging. Magn Reson Med 19:327-332
Moseley I (1995) Imaging the adult brain. J Neurol Neurosurg Psychiatry 58:7-21
Moseley ME, Cohen Y, Mintorovitch J et al (1990a) Early detection of regional cerebral ischemia in cats:
    comparison of diffusion- and T2-weighted MRI and spectroscopy. Magn Reson Med 14:330-346
Moseley ME, Kucharczyk J, Mintorovitch J et al (1990b) Diffusion-weighted MR imaging of acute stroke: cor-
    relation with T2-weighted and magnetic susceptibility-enhanced MR imaging in cats. AJNR 11:423-429
Mueller WM, Yetkin FZ, Hammeke TA et al (1996) Functional magnetic resonance imaging mapping of
    the motor cortex in patients with cerebral tumors. Neurosurgery 39:515-521
Newcombe J, Hawkins CP, Henderson CL et al (1991) Histopathology of multiple sclerosis lesions detected by
    magnetic resonance imaging in unfixed postmortem central nervous system tissue. Brain 114:1013-1023
Ogawa S, Tank DW, Menon R et al (1992) Intrinsic signal changes accompanying sensory stimulation: func-
    tional brain mapping with magnetic resonance imaging. Proc Natl Acad Sci 89:5951-5955
Ojemann JG, Miller JW, Silbergeld DL (1996) Preserved function in brain invaded by tumor. Neurosurgery
    39:253-259
Ordidge RJ, Knight RA, Helpern JA (1991) Magnetization transfer contrast (MTC) in flash MR imaging.
    Magn Reson Imaging 9:889-893
Potchen EJ, Potchen MJ (1991) The imaging of brain function. Positron emission tomography, single-pro-
    ton emission computed tomography and some prospects for magnetic resonance. Invest Radiol 26:258-
    265
Quast MJ, Huang NC, Hillman GR, Kent TA (1993) The evolution of acute stroke recorded by multimodal
    magnetic resonance imaging. Magn Reson Med 11:465-471
Ranjeva JP, Franconi JM, Manelfe C, Berry I (1996) Magnetization transfer in echo-planar imaging MAGMA
    S4:102
Rao SM, Leo GJ, Haughton VM (1989) Correlation of MRI with neuropsychological testing in MS. Neurol-
    ogy 39:161-166
Rao SM, Binder JR, Bandettini PA et al (1993) Functional magnetic resonance imaging of complex human
    movements. Neurology 43:2311-2318
Rao SM, Binder JR, Hammeke TA et al (1995) Somatotopic mapping of the human primary motor cortex
    with functional magnetic resonance imaging. Neurology 45:919-924
Revel M-P, Pons J-C, Lelaidier C, Frydman R, Musset D, Labrune M (1992) Surface coil magnetic resonance
    imaging of the fetal brain. Lancet 340:176
Röther J, Gückel F, Neff W, Schwartz A, Hennerici M (1996) Assessment of regional cerebral blood volume
    in acute human stroke by use of single-slice dynamic susceptibility contrast-enhanced magnetic reso-
    nance imaging. Stroke 27:1088-1093
Sabatini U, Chollet F, Rascol O, Celsis P, Rascol A, Lenzi GL, Marc-Vergnes J-P (1993) Effect of side and rate
    of stimulation on cerebral blood flow changes in motor areas during finger movements in human. J
    Cereb Blood Flow Metab 13:639-645
Sawle GV (1995) Imaging the head: functional imaging. J Neurol Neurosurg Psychiatry 58:132-144
Schad LR, Trost U, Knopp MV, Müller E, Lorenz WJ (1993) Motor cortex stimulation measured by mag-
    netic resonance imaging on a standard 1.5. T clinical scanner. Magn Reson Imaging 11:461-464
Schneider W, Casey BJ, Noll D (1994) Functional MRI mapping of stimulus rate effects across visual process-
    ing stages. Hum Brain Mapp 1:117-133
Sergent J (1994) Brain-imaging studies of cognitive functions. Trends Neurosci 17:221-227
Shaywitz BA, Shaywitz SE, Pugh KR et al (1995a) Sex differences in the functional organization of the brain
    for language. Nature 373:607-609
Shaywitz BA, Pugh KR, Constable RT et al (1995b) Localization of semantic processing using functional
    magnetic resonance imaging. Hum Brain Mapp 2:149-158

Silver NC, Barker GF MacManus DG, Tofts PS, Miller DH (1997) Magnetisation transfer ratio of normal brain white matter: a normative database spanning four decades of life. J Neurol Neurosurg Psychiatry 62:223–228

Simonson TM, Crosby DL, Fisher DJ et al (1994) Echo-planar FLAIR in the evaluation of intracranial lesions. Proceedings, 2nd Annual Meeting of the Society of Magnetic Resonance. San Francisco, pp 522

Skirboll SS, Ojemann GA, Berger MS, Lettich E, Winn HR (1996) Functional cortex and subcortical white matter located within gliomas. Neurosurgery 38:678–685

Sorensen AG, Buonanno FS, Gonzalez RG et al (1996) Hyperacute stroke: evaluation with combined multisection diffusion-weighted and hemodynamically weighted echo-planar MR imaging. Radiology 199:391–401

Thompson AJ, Miller D, Youl B et al (1992) Serial gadolinium-enhanced MRI in relapsing/remitting multiple sclerosis of varying disease duration. Neurology 42:60–63

Thompson RM, Jack CR, Butts K et al (1994) Imaging of cerebral activation at 1.5 T: optimizing a technique for conventional hardware. Radiology 190:873–877

Tomiak M, Rosenblum JD, Prager JM, Metz CE (1994) Magnetization transfer: a potential method to determine the age of multiple sclerosis lesions. Am J Neuroradiol 15:1569–1574

Turner R (1994) Magnetic resonance imaging of brain function. Ann Neurol 35:637–638

Turner R, Jezzard P (1994) Magnetic resonance functional imaging of the brain at 4 T. Magma 2:147–156

Turner R, Jezzard P, Wen H et al (1993) Functional mapping of the human visual cortex at 4 and 1.5 tesla using deoxygenation contrast EPI. Magn Reson Med 29:277–279

Tyszka JM, Grafon ST, Chew W, Woods RP, Colletti PM (1994) Parceling of mesial frontal motor areas during ideation and movement using functional magnetic resonance imaging at 1.5 tesla. Ann Neurol 35:746–749

Ugurbil K, Garwood M, Ellermann J et al (1993) Imaging at high magnetic fields: initial experiences at 4 T. Magn Reson Q 9:259–277

Van Gelderen P, De Vleeschouwer MHM, DesPres D, Pekar J, Van Zijl PCM, Moonen CTM (1994) Water diffusion and acute stroke. Magn Reson Med 31:154

Villringer A, Rosen B, Belliveau JW et al (1988) Dynamic imaging with lanthanide chelates in normal brain: contrast due to magnetic susceptibility effects. Magn Reson Med 6:164–174

Warach S, Li W, Ronthal M, Edelman RR (1992a) Acute cerebral ischemia: evaluation with dynamic contrast-enhanced MR imaging and MR angiography. Radiology 182:41–47

Warach S, Chien D, Li W, Ronthal M, Edelman RR (1992b) Fast magnetic resonance diffusion-weighted imaging of acute human stroke. Neurology 42:1717–1723

Warach S, Gaa J, Siewert B, Wielopolski P, Edelman RR (1995) Acute human stroke studied by whole brain echo planar diffusion-weighted magnetic resonance imaging. Ann Neurol 37:231–241

Warach S, Dashe JF, Edelman RR (1996) Clinical outcome in ischemic stroke predicted by early diffusion-weighted and perfusion magnetic resonance imaging: a preliminary analysis. J Cereb Blood Flow Metab 16:53–59

Weiller C, Chollet F, Friston KJ et al (1992) Functional reorganization of the brain in recovery from striatocapsular infarction in man. Ann Neurol 31:463–472

Welch KMA, Windham J, Knight RA et al (1995) A model to predict the histopathology of human stroke using diffusion and T2-weighted magnetic resonance imaging. Stroke 26:1983–1989

Wenstrom KD, Williamson RA, Weiner CP, Sipes SL, Yuh WTC (1991) Magnetic resonance imaging of fetuses with intracranial defects. Obstet Gynecol 77:529–532

Wolff SD, Balaban RS (1989) Magnetization transfer contrast (MTC) and tissue water proton relaxation in vivo. Magn Reson Med 10:135–144

Wolff SD, Balaban RS (1994) Magnetization transfer imaging: practical aspects and clinical applications. Radiology 192:593–599

Wolff SD, Eng J, Balaban RS (1991) Magnetization transfer contrast: method for improving contrast in gradient recalled-echo images. Radiology 179:133–137

Wood RP, Cherry SR, Mazziotta JC (1992) Rapid automated algorithm for aligning and reslicing PET images. J Comput Assist Tomogr 115:565–587

Yousry TA, Schmid UD, Jassoy AG et al (1995) Topography of the cortical motor hand area: prospective study with functional MR functional imaging and direct motor mapping at surgery. Radiology 195:23–29

Zimmerman RA, Girard N (1995) Magnetization transfer in the evaluation of patients with tuberous sclerosis. Radiology 197(P):306

3   Ultrafast Magnetic Resonance Imaging of the Heart

H.J. Lamb, J. Doornbos, and A. de Roos

1   Introduction

Magnetic resonance imaging (MRI) provides an excellent tool for the evaluation of the heart. A wide array of fast MR techniques have become available for examining coronary artery anatomy and flow, cardiac function, myocardial perfusion, and metabolism. Cardiac MRI methods may be divided into conventional methods, such as spin-echo sequences, and fast-imaging methods, including echo-planar-imaging (EPI) and fast gradient-echo sequences. The acquisition and display of the information available by these techniques within a single comprehensive imaging session may provide a useful test for guiding patient management in a cost-effective manner. Until now most studies have focused on the feasibility and optimization of MR technology for assessing the heart and its most significant disease processes. Further technological progress in acquiring and processing the multitude of data obtained during an MR examination is still required.

The clinical role of MRI is expected to increase steadily for the evaluation of ischemic heart disease, which depends on the implementation of ultrafast MRI techniques. This chapter addresses the role of fast MRI for evaluating myocardial perfusion and function.

2   MRI in Myocardial Ischemia

2.1   Introduction

Conventional MRI allows identification of the region of acute myocardial ischemia without the aid of MR contrast agents (Wisenberg et al. 1988; Johnston et al. 1989). Both T1 and T2 relaxation parameters may be altered in the area of ischemia due to the presence of myocardial edema. MRI based on T2-weighting has been advocated to detect acute myocardial infarction, to evaluate infarct size, and to assess healing patterns in patients following reperfusion (Johns et al. 1990). However, visualizing myocardial infarction on T2-weighted MR sequences relies on the accumulation of free water within the infarcted region, which may take several hours to develop. In addition, T2-weighted spin-echo sequences may be hampered by motion artifacts, limiting its value for evaluating myocardial infarction (Matheijssen et al. 1991). Furthermore, non-contrast-enhanced MR techniques provide no information on tissue perfusion.

The newly developed MRI techniques allow very fast or even real-time kinematic imaging of the ventricles (Heid 1997; Kerr et al. 1997; Stuber et al. 1997; Yang et al. 1997) and visualization of myocardial perfusion following the administration of contrast agents.

2.2   Review of Clinical Applications of MRI in Ischemic Heart Disease

Until recently most contrast-enhanced MR studies in patients with acute and subacute myocardial infarction were performed with the aid of gadolinium-based compounds during the equilibrium phase using relatively slow imaging techniques (e.g., T1-weighted spin-echo imaging). Fast imaging techniques have now become available for high temporal resolution imaging of the heart during the first pass of intravenously administered contrast media (Atkinson et al. 1990).

Most clinical experience has been obtained with extracellular agents such as gadolinium-DTPA, which can be safely used in patients with coronary artery disease and generally provide a better image quality than unenhanced T2-weighted approaches (Matheijssen et al. 1991). The delayed contrast enhancement in the ischemic region is probably caused by differences in wash-in and wash-out of gadolinium-DTPA between the normal and ischemic myocardium. In the acutely damaged myocardium the increased accumulation of gadolinium-DTPA may be related to a number of factors: decreased blood flow, increased tissue blood volume, expansion of the extracellular space, increased permeability of the capillaries, and ingrowth of granulation tissue. By 10–15 min after gadolinium-DTPA administration it has largely washed out from the normal myocardium, whereas it is retained in the infarcted zone. This suggests that contrast-enhanced MRI in acute myocardial infarction has an optimal time window approximately 15 min after contrast medium administration ("hot spot" imaging; de Roos et al. 1989; Higgins et al. 1993).

Gadolinium-DTPA has no cellular uptake and is excreted with a relatively short half-live time by glomerular filtration. Eichstaedt et al. (1986) demonstrated that significant infarct enhancement occurs in the acute (days 5–10 after infarct onset) and subacute (first 3 weeks) phases but not in the chronic (after 3 weeks) phase. This observation suggests that optimal infarct enhancement occurs during injury of cell membranes when ingrowth of granulation tissue plays an important role. In line with these initial observations several other studies have reported marked infarct enhancement in the acute and subacute phases of infarct healing with a maximal effect within the first week after infarction (Nishimura et al. 1989a; van Dijkman et al. 1991).

The use of gadolinium-DTPA improves visualization of both reperfused and nonreperfused infarcts (de Roos et al. 1989). Signal intensity ratios between infarcted and normal myocardium appear to plateau 15–20 min after contrast administration. Infarct enhancement patterns can be observed which may reflect the presence or absence of reperfusion. Uniform, homogeneous enhancement of the infarcted region may indicate successful reperfusion, whereas peripheral enhancement may be a marker of nonreperfusion. In addition, the early dynamics of infarct enhancement may signify the presence or absence of reperfusion. Reperfused

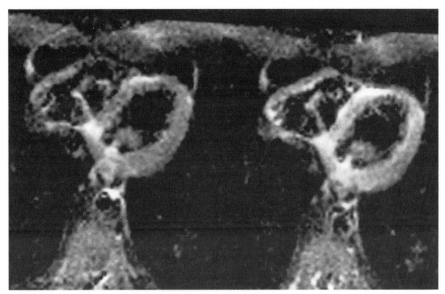

Fig. 1. Axial segmented (four shots interleaved) spin-echo EPI images acquired before and after administration of paramagnetic contrast (Gd-DTPA 0.1 mmol/kg). Each 2D spin-echo EPI data set consists of six contiguous axial sections acquired in a gated fashion over two heart beats. Contrast enhancement of the entire myocardium can be clearly demonstrated. The sequence is sufficiently T1-weighted to result in an actual signal increase in the myocardium following the administration of paramagnetic contrast. (Courtesy of Dr. J.F. Debatin)

infarcts reveal an early and more pronounced degree of enhancement than nonreperfused infarcts (van Rossum et al. 1990). Gadolinium-DTPA enhanced spin-echo MRI has also been used to measure the area of acute myocardial infarction (Nishimura et al. 1989b; de Roos et al. 1990). The average size of reperfused infarcts proved to be significantly smaller than that of nonreperfused infarcts [8% ± 5% versus 15% ± 4% of left ventricular (LV) mass]. This approach may be useful to assess the effect of reperfusion therapies on infarct size.

Recently Davis et al. (1995) applied spin-echo EPI for fast imaging of the myocardial wall using gadolinium-DTPA (Fig. 1). Fast MRI can also be applied to visualize the sodium content of myocardial tissue. Kim et al. (1997) studied dogs and rabbits after acute myocardial infarction and showed increased sodium content in reperfused myocardial tissue after occlusion.

2.3   Myocardial Perfusion Imaging

2.3.1   Image Acquisition

Coronary atherosclerosis is the most common underlying cause of coronary artery disease. Atherosclerosis becomes manifest when coronary artery narrowing results in reduced coronary flow and the development of myocardial ischemia.

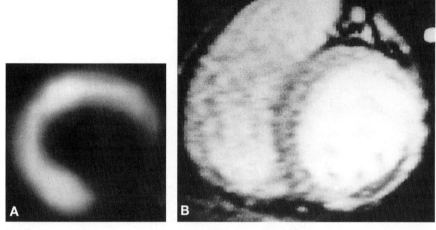

Fig. 2A, B. Images of a patient with cardiac infarction showing hypoperfusion of the LV. A Thallium scintigram showing a perfusion defect in the posterior wall. (B), First-pass ultrafast MR image obtained immediately after injection of Gd-GTPA, showing a subendocardial hypoperfused dark area in the posterior wall which corresponds to the affected region in (A). The normal myocardium has enhanced signal due to increased T1-relaxation after administration of the contrast agent (Courtesy Dr. E.A. Zerhouni)

Coronary flow is controlled by constriction and dilatation of the coronary resistance vessels. Measuring myocardial perfusion is of prime importance in assessing the functional significance of the morphology of coronary obstructions. Flow information is useful for risk stratification in patients with suspected coronary artery disease and to determine whether chest pain is related to obstructive coronary artery disease, and in patients following acute myocardial infarction. Although the extent of acute myocardial infarction can be estimated from T2-weighted spin-echo MR images, delineation of the area at jeopardy distal to coronary artery stenoses requires the use of contrast media.

Ultrafast MRI offers the opportunity to acquire dynamic information related to the passage of a MR contrast medium through the myocardium and thus provides an indirect measure of myocardial perfusion. MR contrast media are required as a perfusion marker to evaluate first-pass transit after bolus administration of the agent. Ultrafast MRI consists of an inversion prepulse followed by a gradient-echo sequence with very short repetition times and echo times to obtain a T1-weighted image in a fraction of the cardiac cycle (Fig. 2; Atkinson et al. 1990; Manning et al. 1991; van Rugge et al. 1991). Feasibility studies initially demonstrated the first-pass transit of gadolinium-DTPA through the cardiac compartments and LV myocardium after peripheral bolus injection of the contrast medium.

A limitation of the ultrafast technique is that only one or a few tomographic sections are obtained during first-pass perfusion. Myocardial perfusion studies

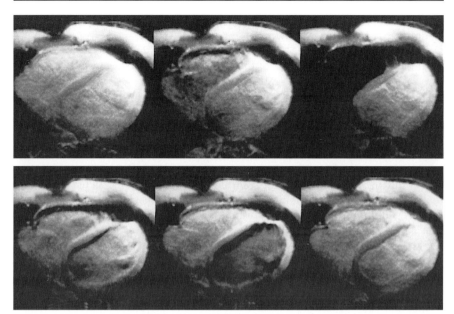

Fig. 3. Segmented EPI (two shots interleaved) images depicting the T2-shortening effect of paramagnetic contrast (Gd-DTPA 0.05 mmol/kg) passing through the cardiac chambers and into the myocardium. Each 2D data set consisting of six contiguous 10 mm thick slices is acquired in the transverse plane in a gated fashion, every two heart beats. Reflecting T2* weighting of the EPI sequence, there is darkening of the blood as it passes through the cardiac chambers. The interface of the environments of strongly different magnetic susceptibility causes artifacts which can falsify assesment of myocardial perfusion with this technique. (Courtesy of Dr. J.F. Debatin)

both at rest and under stress become clinically useful when images can be obtained in a multislice mode instead of the single-slice acquisition which has been used until now. Recently methods were developed to image several levels of the LV during the first pass of perfusion markers (Fischer et al. 1997). Figure 3 displays images obtained with an EPI sequence; this example also notes a potential pitfall of perfusion imaging with paramagnctic contrast agents.

2.3.2 Flow Quantitation

Although attempts are made to quantify perfusion in absolute terms, the accurate assessment of relative perfusion may provide clinical useful information. Absolute quantification of myocardial perfusion is hampered by several prerequisites which must be fulfilled (Wood et al. 1994), including:
a) the contrast medium is mixed completely and uniformly with the blood,
b) the volume of the contrast medium is negligible to the volume of the vasculature,
c) the indicator does not affect the hemodynamics of flow,
d) the indicator does not affect the vascular equilibrium,

e) the relationship between the change in signal intensity and the concentration of the indicator is known,

f) recirculation is negligible, and

g) there is no extravascular loss of the indicator during first pass.

Normal and ischemic myocardium differ in perfusion or instantaneous blood volume, which results in a difference in the local concentration of the contrast medium between normal and abnormal tissue. Fast gradient-echo or echo-planar MR techniques can be used to monitor the passage of contrast media through the central circulation and to follow the first pass through the myocardium as a marker for regional blood volume or perfusion. Signal intensity versus time curves during the first passage of contrast media can be constructed as an estimate of regional myocardial blood flow. However, the use of extracellular agents such as gadolinium-DTPA is not optimal for myocardial perfusion imaging because these agents are not confined to one tissue compartment. As a consequence the accumulation of gadolinium-DTPA and other extracellular contrast agents in the myocardium depends not only on tissue blood volume and blood flow but also on the intravascular and interstitial distribution volumes as well as the permeability of the capillaries (Wilke et al. 1993). It is estimated that approximately 50% of the injected dose of gadolinium-DTPA is cleared from the capillaries during the first pass through the myocardium.

Unfortunately, the relationship between myocardial signal intensity following the administration of extracellular contrast and the concentration of the contrast agent is complex, limiting the possibilities for absolute quantification of perfusion. In addition, first-pass myocardial perfusion studies require a rapid bolus injection within 2 s and an imaging sequence with a high temporal resolution of at least one image per heart beat to capture the transit of the contrast agent through the myocardium, thereby avoiding problems caused by recirculation of the contrast medium (Wilke et al. 1993; Keijer et al. 1995). A potential confounding factor that may preclude reliable myocardial perfusion imaging is the methodology of contrast medium administration. It has been noted that the ventricular signal intensity versus time curves depend on the injection site (peripheral bolus injection versus injection through a catheter placed in the right atrium) and bolus concentration (Keijer et al. 1995). In spite of the experimental and theoretical difficulties mentioned above Jerosch-Herold et al. (1997) recently developed an approach for absolute flow quantification (in milliliter per gram per minute) in the myocardium.

2.3.3   Potential Applications

Despite a number of limitations MR perfusion imaging has successfully been applied in patients with healed myocardial infarcts to identify the scar as a relative perfusion defect (van Rugge et al. 1992a) and also for detecting perfusion-related abnormalities in the myocardium distal to coronary artery stenoses with more than 80% luminal narrowing (Manning et al. 1991). Time versus intensity curves reveal lower peak signal intensity and lower upslope of signal increase distal to significant coronary artery stenoses than normally perfused myocardium. These perfusion abnormalities may restore to normal after successful reperfusion therapy (Manning et al. 1991). These results were achieved employing fast gradient-recalled echo (GRE) sequences. These allow the acquisition of only one or two sections through the heart. Multishot EPI sequences allow coverage of the entire heart, but image quality and contrast have to date limited their use.

2.3.4   Stress MR Perfusion

Dipyridamole stress can be applied to reveal perfusion defects distal to coronary artery stenoses which may not be detected under resting conditions (Matheijssen et al. 1996). Dipyridamole acts as a coronary vasodilator (van Rugge et al. 1992b). Its dilating action has not been fully elucidated but appears to be related to the increased plasma level of endogenous adenosine, a potent coronary arteriolar vasodilator. In patients with significant coronary artery stenoses, the vascular bed distal to the stenosis is somewhat dilated to promote normal resting flow. Therefore severe stenosis results in an exhausted flow reserve, and dipyridamole administration does not result in further vasodilatation of the stenosed vessel. In contrast, normal coronary arteries retain their full capacity to vasodilate. Hence a regional flow heterogeneity or perfusion maldistribution between normal and ischemic myocardium becomes evident.

Pennell et al. (1990a) were the first to report the results of dipyridamole stress MRI in patients with coronary artery disease. Reversible wall motion abnormalities were detected in only 67% of patients with reversible thallium perfusion defects, indicating that dipyridamole is not ideally suited to induce wall motion abnormalities. Several studies have shown the feasibility of dipyridamole stress MRI for detecting perfusion abnormalities related to coronary artery disease with a sensitivity, specificity, and accuracy of 65%, 76%, and 74%, respectively (Pennell et al. 1990b; Eichenberger et al. 1994; Matheijssen et al. 1996). Matheijssen et al. (1996) used double-level MR perfusion imaging in patients with documented single-vessel coronary artery disease using gadolinium-DTPA as a perfusion marker before and after dipyridamole infusion. A good correlation between MR-defined perfusion defects during dipyridamole hyperemia and tomographic technetium-99m sestaMIBI (SPECT) imaging was found. Quantitative analysis of signal intensity versus time curves obtained with MRI revealed that the slope of the signal intensity curve following bolus injection of gadolinium-DTPA correctly identified perfusion abnormalities (Matheijssen et al. 1996). In a similar study Dendale et al. (1997) showed that MR perfusion imaging using an ultrafast gradient-echo sequence distinguishes between open and closed infarct-related arteries by identifying myocardial regions with slower wash-in and reduced wash-out properties.

Myocardial viability may also be studied by fast MRI tissue tagging, as shown by Kramer et al. (1997). In a study of 13 patients they analyzed myocardial circumferential shortening with MRI tissue tagging before and during low-dose dobutamine infusion. A quantitatively normal circumferential shortening response to dobutamine within disfunctional myocardium early after infarction proved to be a sensitive predictor of quantitative improvement in function as measured with MRI 8 weeks after the myocardial infarction (Kramer et al. 1997).

2.4   MR Angiography of the Coronary Arteries

2.4.1   Image Acquisition

The techniques for coronary artery MRI are in an experimental phase and require further technical development. MR angiography is used routinely in many centers for evaluation of the carotid arteries, intracerebral, and abdominal vasculature. MR angiography of the coronary arteries, however, is technically more demanding due to the relatively small vessel size, their complex three-dimensional anatomy, and their constantly changing position within the thoracic cavity due to cardiac and respiration motion (van der Wall et al. 1995).

GRE techniques have been used to image the proximal coronary arteries in healthy subjects (Wang et al. 1991). Three-dimensional MR angiograms were constructed by stacking two-dimensional planar images (Cho et al. 1991). Faster methods such as EPI (Stehling et al. 1987), and fast spiral EPI (Meyer et al. 1992)

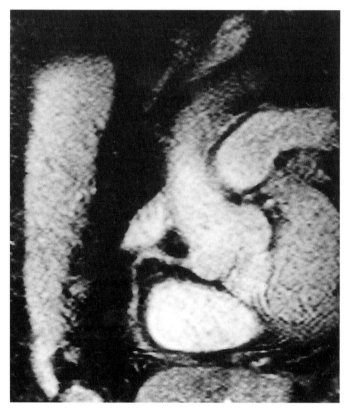

Fig. 4. Coronary MR angiogram, obtained during a breath-hold. The right coronary artery is clearly visible. The image was obtained using a fast gradient-echo segmented k-space sequence, with fat suppression. (Courtesy of Philips Medical Systems)

have also been proposed. Until now the best results on commercially available scanners have been obtained using an ultrafast GRE technique during periods of breath-holding introduced by Edelman et al. (1991). Breath-holding is essential to avoid excessive blurring from respiratory motion. Fat suppression is used to improve contrast between coronary arteries and surrounding epicardial fat. Transverse sections permit assessment of the left main, left anterior descending, and proximal right coronary arteries, whereas oblique imaging sections are best for depicting the left circumflex artery and the more distal segments of the right coronary artery (Fig. 4). As many as 20–30 interleaved segments are acquired and scan times (breath-holding periods) are 15–18 s for each image acquisition. Sequentially obtained slices (2D) or slabs (3D) may be processed by the maximum intensity projection to allow an overview of the area under investigation (Fig. 5).

In an initial study by Manning et al. (1993a) 19 normal subjects and six patients with coronary artery disease were imaged using this technique. Imaging time was approximately 45 min. Mean vessel diameter ranged from 2.6 mm (left circumflex artery) to 6.2 mm (left main coronary artery) which was well correlated with quantitative contrast angiography. Mean visualized vessel length ranged from 8 mm (left main coronary artery) to 122 mm (right coronary artery).

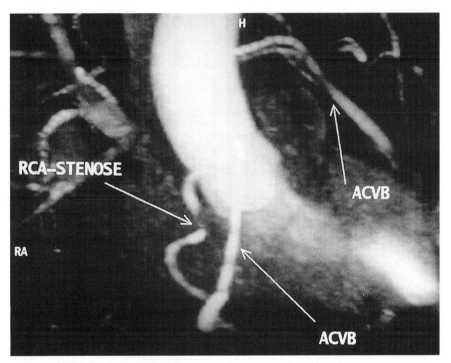

Fig. 5. Maximum intensity projection of a series of coronary MR angiograms showing a stenosis of the right coronary artery (*RCA*). Aortocoronary venous bypass grafts (*ACVB*) are clearly visible. (Courtesy of Dr. A. von Smekal)

Occluded vessels appeared as absent flow signal distal to the occlusion and high-grade stenoses appeared as signal loss in the area of stenosis with visualization of the vessel distally. In a subsequent study Manning et al. (1993b) compared MR coronary angiography with conventional angiography: the sensitivity and specificity of MR coronary angiography, as compared with conventional angiography, for correctly identifying individual vessels with at least 50% angiographic stenoses were 90% and 92%, respectively. The corresponding positive and negative predictive values were 85% and 95%, respectively. The sensitivity and specificity of the technique were 100% and 100%, respectively, for the left main coronary artery, 87% and 92% for the left anterior descending artery, 71% and 90% for the left circumflex coronary artery, and 100% and 78% for the right coronary artery. Pennell et al. (1993) studied 21 healthy controls and 5 patients with coronary artery disease using a similar segmented k-space gradient-echo imaging

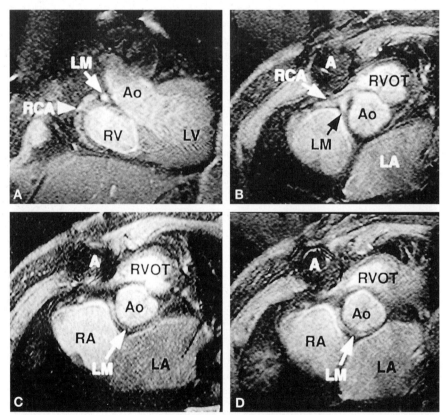

Fig. 6A–D. MR angiograms of a patient with an anomalous course of the left main (*LM*) coronary artery. A oblique view; B, C, D contiguous transverse images. The left main stem courses behind the aorta (*Ao*). *LV*, Left ventricle; *LA*, left atrium; *RVOT*, right ventricular outflow tract; *RCA*, right coronary artery; *RV* right ventricle. The images were obtained using a fast gradient-echo segmented k-space sequence, with fat suppression. (Courtesy of Dr. H.J. Vliegen)

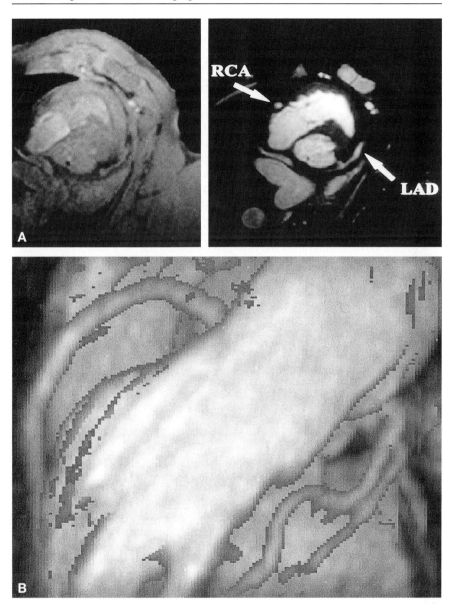

Fig. 7A, B. Application of the intravascular MR contrast agent Gd-BSA. (**A**) Pre contrast (*left*) and post contrast (*right*) transverse T1-weigthed image of a pig heart. The right coronary artery (*RCA*) and the left anterior descending coronary artery (*LAD*) are indicated. (**B**) Closest vessel projection of the complete 3D dataset. (Courtesy of M.B.M. Hofman, St. Louis). See Hofmann MBM et al., 5th Scientific Meeting of ISMRM, Vancouver 1997, p442.

technique. A complete image is obtained in 16 cardiac cycles during one breath-holding. The left main stem (95%), left anterior descending coronary artery (91%), and right coronary artery were identified in all subjects, but identification of the left circumflex coronary artery proved more difficult (76%). A good correlation was found between measurements made by MRI and contrast coronary angiography.

A limitation of MR angiography is the requirement of a regular sinus rhythm and the need for breath-holding during 15–18 s. To overcome the latter a breath-holding strategy was introduced that requires only a 1-s breath-hold in every 4 s (Doyle et al. 1993). Frequent ventricular extrasystoles, however, can also result in degradation of the quality of the image. The present spatial resolution and loss of signal due to turbulence preclude accurate prediction of the severity of stenosis. Hope can be based on recent advances showing high-resolution MR angiograms of the coronary arteries obtained during a (relatively long) breath-hold, following interactive localization of the scan plane (Meyer et al. 1997).

Coronary MR angiography has also been shown to be very useful in detecting and confirming a suspected congenitally anomalous course of the coronary arteries. The proximal 4–5 cm of the right coronary artery, the left main coronary artery, and the left anterior descending coronary artery can be visualized (Doorey et al. 1994; Duerinckx et al. 1995; Post et al. 1995; Vliegen et al. 1997; see Fig. 6).

To avoid the need for breath-holding, navigator echoes have been succesfully applied to MR coronary angiography (Oshinski et al. 1996; Post et al. 1996).

New intravascular contrast agents may play a role in extending the possibilities of MR coronary angiography (Fig. 7). The application of contrast agents in MR angiography extends the choice of imaging sequences to methods that are not specifically sensitive to inflow of magnetically unsaturated blood in the image plane.

2.4.2 Coronary Flow Reserve

Poncelet et al. (1993) demonstrated the potential of echo-planar MRI to detect flow velocity changes in coronary arteries during isometric exercise. Flow velocity in coronary arteries measured using MRI was shown to be in agreement with flow values obtained with intracoronary Doppler flow measurements (Furber et al. 1997). These findings suggest the utility of this technique to evaluate coronary flow reserve. Sakuma et al. (1996) showed promising results concerning the noninvasive determination of coronary flow reserve. Breath-hold velocity-encoded cine MRI provided reproducible assessment of coronary flow reserve in healthy vounteers (Fig. 8A,8B). They also applied the protocol to patients with coronary stenosis (Fig. 8C). MR flow measurements showed a significant difference between normal healthy subjects and the patients studied concerning the coronary flow reserve. It is thought that, if all these techniques continue to progress, MRI will become useful for screening the major coronary arteries for significant coronary artery disease. The promising results regarding coronary flow measurements with MRI have recently been corroborated in several reports (Davis et al. 1997; Globits et al. 1997; Grist et al. 1997).

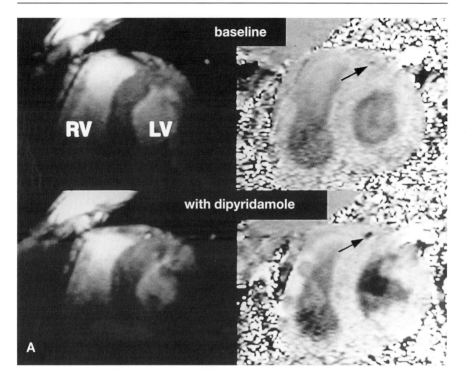

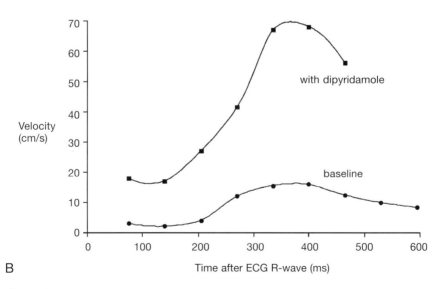

Fig. 8A, B

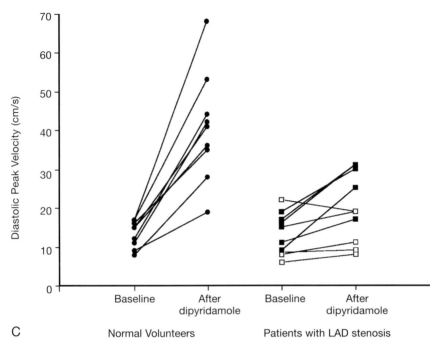

Fig. 8A–C. A short axis view of the LV in a healthy volunteer. *Left*, magnitude images; *right*, velocity-encoded images. Images were obtained before (upper panel) and after administration of the coronary vasodilator dipyridamole (*arrows*, left anterior descending artery). (**B**) Flow velocities measured in the coronary artery (*LAD*, see *arrows* in (**A**) during the R-R interval. *Lower trace*, rest situation; *upper trace*, stress situation. Note the significant increase in flow velocity induced by dipyridamole (see also ref. Sakuma 1996). (**C**) Diastolic peak velocity (*DPV*) measured by fast velocity encoded MRI at baseline state and after dipyridamole administration. DPV changed substantially in the normal volunteers, from 13.5 ± 3.3 at baseline to 41.9 ± 13.2 after dipyridamole infusion. The resulting coronary flow reserve (*CFR*) was 3.1 in the normal volunteers. In patients with LAD stenosis DPV was only slightly increased from 13.1 ± 6.1 at baseline to 20.5 ± 8.9 after dipyridamole infusion. The calculated CFR was 1.6 in these patients. Note the difference between patients with an LAD stenosis ≤ 75% (*filled squares*) and patients with an LAD stenosis ≥ 75% (*open squares*). (Courtesy of Dr. C.B. Higgins, Dr. H. Sakuma)

3   Myocardial Function

3.1   Introduction

Regional abnormalities of contraction and relaxation are early and sensitive markers of disturbed ventricular performance in patients with ischemic heart disease. These regional function abnormalities may become evident only under stress conditions due to stress-induced ischemia, whereas global ventricular function remains normal as reflected by normal end-systolic and end-diastolic volumes, stroke volumes, and ejection fraction. Global ventricular function is maintained owing to augmented motion of normal segments of the myocardium, which compensate for decreased regional function in ischemic segments. When ischemic disease becomes more severe, regional dysfunction may become manifest also under resting conditions.

3.2   Wall Motion Analysis

Gradient-echo MRI can be used for the analysis of global and regional cardiac function (Sechtem et al. 1987). Both abnormal wall motion and more specifically abnormal wall thickening indicate diminished regional myocardial function. Pflugfelder et al. (1988) studied 13 normal subjects and 15 patients with coronary artery disease by gradient-echo MRI to document and quantify regional LV wall motion abnormalities. Abnormal wall motion was observed in 40–90 segments in patients with coronary artery disease, which was well correlated with results of echocardiography and contrast ventriculography. Overall systolic wall thickening in the normal subjects was 48% ± 28%. In patients, in the normal segments (43% ± 31%) were easily differentiated from hypokinetic (6% ± 18%) akinetic (-4% ± 24%), and dyskinetic zones (-13% ± 25%). Thus the absence of systolic wall thickening proved a highly specific marker of regional myocardial dysfunction. Lotan et al. (1989) studied 59 patients with suspected coronary artery disease with both gradient-echo MRI and biplane cineangiography. In the right anterior oblique view there was agreement in 96% of 275 segments, and in the left anterior oblique view in 92% of segments. Holman et al. (1997) proposed a method to quantify the extent of the myocardial infarction in 3D by using the improved centerline method. The results were well correlated with enzymatically obtained information on the extent of myocardial infarction.

Fast MR methods have been recently introduced to study wall motion characteristics (Szolar et al. 1996). Szolar et al. showed, in an experimental study in dogs, that contractile dysfunction is in close agreement with myocardial perfusion defects obtained simultaneously in the same animals, and they concluded that fast MRI may be useful to monitor postischemic myocardial abnormalities following thrombolytic therapy as well as the response to pharmacological interventions.

Wall motion may also be assessed directly using velocity-encoded gradient-echo sequences. Wedeen (1992) described techniques to measure wall motion and local strain rates and showed local instantaneous strain rates in the human LV myocardium to be quantitatively consistent with known transmural average values of myocardial strain. The accuracy of these motion tracking techniques was confirmed by Pelc et al. (1994), who used fast phase contrast techniques. LV circumferential shortening measured by velocity mapping appears be a valuable parameter as studied preinfarct and postinfarct in a canine model (Constable et al. 1994). The combination of breath-hold imaging with tagging and velocity-encoding sequences has made the measurement of myocardial wall motion in patients a simple and reproducible examination. These methods enable quantification of the severity and extent of regional heart wall motion abnormalities

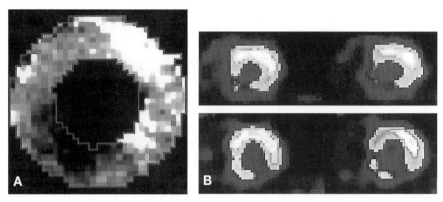

Fig. 9A–B.   (**A**), MR image of the radial velocity of the myocardium measured in a polar co-ordinate system centered in the LV. The observed slice is located 3 cm from the base of the heart in a patient with a posterior infarction acquired at 90 ms after the R wave of the ECG. In the MR image outward motion is dark and inward motion is bright. (**B**), Tl-201 scintigram of the same patient. The scintigrams represent two parallel sections during two time frames in sys-tole. The infarcted region is akinetic or even dyskinetic. (Courtesy of Dr. J. Hennig)

both at rest and during stress. A review of these methods was recently provided by McVeigh (1996). Figure 9 displays the value of myocardial velocity mapping in a patient with a posterior myocardial infarction, as obtained with a black blood prepared segmented gradient-echo sequence (Hennig and Schneider 1997).

3.3   Correction for Respiratory Motion

Conventional GRE techniques are characterized by relatively long acquisition times which make them sensitive to respiratory motion. Respiratory motion is the main cause of degradation of image quality, resulting in relatively high vari-ability of measurements of functional parameters (Pattynama et al. 1993). Since GRE techniques require several hundred heart beats to produce a movie loop of a slice with sufficient image quality, breath-holding is not feasible.

These limitations can be overcome by using fast MRI techniques such as seg-mented k-space GRE sequences (Edelman et al. 1990) and EPI (Mansfield 1977). These techniques allow real-time or nearly real-time visualization of cardiac func-tion during a breath-hold (Sakuma et al. 1993; Baldy et al. 1994; Hunter et al. 1994; Unterweger et al. 1994). EPI represents the fastest clinically useful imaging technique and is well suited for monitoring cardiac motion (Edelman et al. 1994). EPI can operate as a single-shot technique as well as a segmented k-space se-quence by multishot EPI (Butts et al. 1993, 1994; McKinnon 1993; Davis et al. 1995). Multishot EPI is less affected by susceptibility artifacts and poses fewer demands on gradient performance than the single-shot technique (Edelman et al. 1994). Figure 10 shows an application of real-time EPI of the heart. Figure 11 is an ex-ample of an EPI sequence gated over four heart beats.

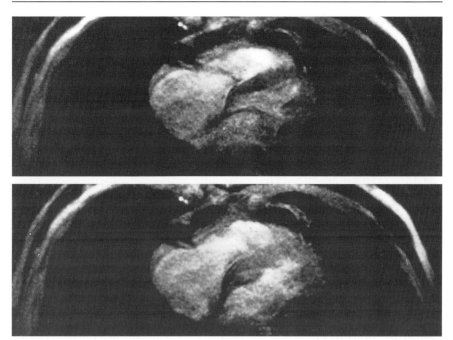

Fig. 10. Segmented EPI (four shots interleaved) acquisition of the heart demonstrating the mitral valve in open and closed position. The images are acquired over 84 ms each. No gating is necessary in this mode (Courtesy of Dr. J.F. Debatin)

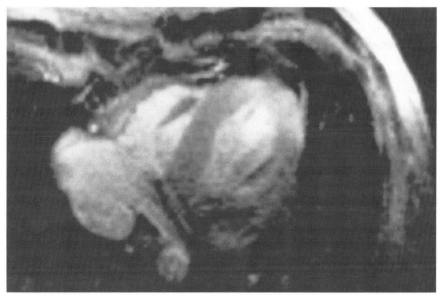

Fig. 11. Segmented EPI (four shots interleaved) image traversing the heart. The image was acquired gated over four heart beats. Image quality is sufficient to delineate papillary muscles as well as the coronary sinus (Courtesy of Dr. J.F. Debatin)

3.3.1   Breath-Hold Segmented EPI

Until recently EPI was available only on special or modified MRI systems (Rzedzian and Pykett 1987; Unterweger et al. 1994). The majority of previous applications of EPI to evaluate heart function were limited to unangulated transaxial or coronal acquisitions (Davis et al. 1994, 1995; Unterweger et al. 1994; Wetter et al. 1995). LV measurements based on EPI images were obtained for end-systolic volume, end-diastolic volume, ejection fraction, stroke volume, and cardiac output (Hunter et al. 1994; Unterweger et al. 1994). Recently multishot EPI was implemented on commercially available MR scanners, allowing double-oblique imaging of the LV in the short-axis orientation. Consequently EPI was recently applied to determine LV mass and diastolic function (Lamb et al. 1996). This MRI study was performed using a standard 1.5-T MRI system without modification of gradient coils (ACS-NT15, Gyroscan).

The imaging protocol (Lamb et al. 1996) to acquire basic functional LV parameters was as follows; Based on images in the transverse plane (Fig. 12) right anterior oblique equivalent (two-chamber view) images were centered through the apex of the LV to intersect the mitral valve plane (Fig. 13). To acquire a four-chamber view a slice was positioned to transect the apex of the LV on the diastolic and systolic two-chamber images and was centered low on the mitral valve plane (Fig. 14). Planned on the diastolic and systolic two-chamber and four-chamber images, the heart was imaged from apex to base with ten imaging levels in the short-axis orientation (Fig. 15). All ten sections were imaged with conventional GRE and with EPI during the same 45-min MR examination, including patient positioning and patient instruction time. Excitation slice thickness was 8 mm, with an intersection gap of 1–2 mm, depending on heart size. Field of view was 40 × 40 cm. Multishot echo-planar gradient-echo was performed with a maximum gradient amplitude of 15 mT/m, which could be reached in 0.9 ms. Consequently the slew rate was 16.7 mT m^{-1} ms^{-1} for the x, y, and z gradient axes. TE was 11 ms with a resulting echo spacing of (11/4=) 2.75 ms, the time to measure a single k-space line. The EPI sequence was not a partial echo technique; no data averaging and no fat suppression was applied. Images were obtained as a 112 × 128 matrix and were reconstructed to 256 × 256-pixel images. Using this multishot EPI technique seven lines in k-space (total was 112 lines) can be obtained after a single excitation by a 30° radio frequency pulse, whereas single-shot EPI techniques acquire all k-space lines following a single α-pulse (Davis et al. 1995; Wetter et al. 1995). Each section level was scanned separately during a single breath-hold in expiration with a maximal duration of 15 s.

This study proved that double-oblique, fast evaluation of LV mass and systolic and diastolic function is possible using a multishot EPI technique with breath-holding on a standard MR scanner. EPI allows acquisition of MR images covering the entire heart in about 7 min with a 2.5-min actual acquisition time. EPI-derived measurements are at least as accurate as data obtained from the more time-consuming conventional GRE imaging (Lamb et al. 1996; Fig. 15). Absence of respiratory artifacts contributes to more reproducible and faster detection of endocardial and epicardial borders of the LV, thereby improving functional evaluation of the heart (Figs. 16, 17).

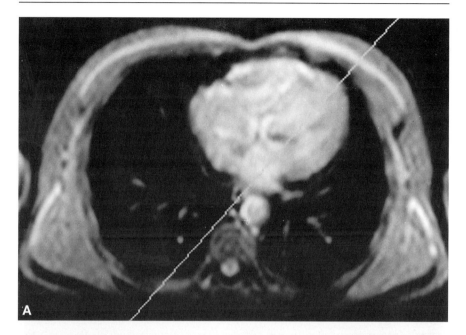

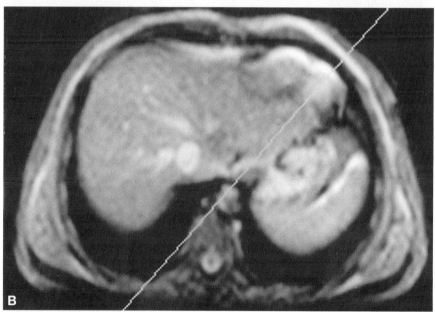

Fig. 12. Transverse survey images obtained with segmented EPI during a 10-s breath-hold. The two-chamber view is planned by positioning the center of a slice in the middle of the mitral valve on a transverse image at the mitral valve level of the heart (**A**) and thereafter by angulating the slice through the apex in the lowest transverse survey image to show blood signal (**B**). The two-chamber view is shown in Figure 13

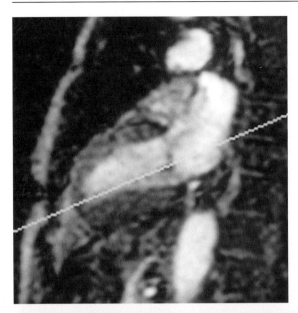

Fig. 13. Two-chamber view in end-systole, acquired with multishot EPI during a 10-s breath-hold. During this time 23 images were obtained to provide a cine movie loop of the cardiac contraction. On this image and the accompanying end-diastolic image (not shown) the four-chamber view was planned. The slice center was positioned just below the center of the mitral valve in the end-systolic image and angulated through the apex. The four chamber view is shown in Figure 14

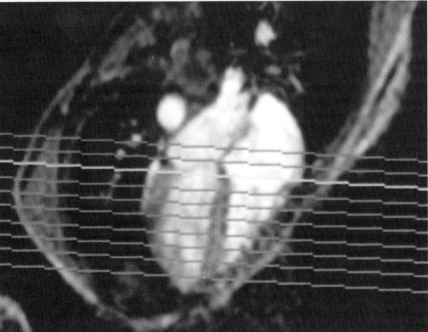

Fig. 14. Four-chamber view in end-diastole and end-systole, acquired with segmented EPI during a 10-s breath-hold. From the end-diastolic and end-systolic images in the two-chamber view and four-chamber view the short-axis scan was planned. Slices were positioned perpendicular to the long axis of the LV, which is from the midmitral point to the apex. The resulting short-axis view is shown in Figure 15

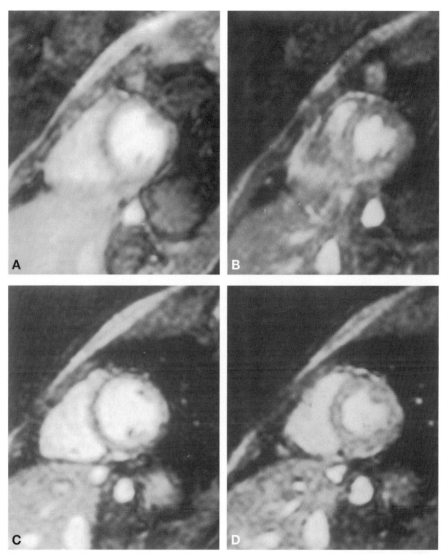

Fig. 15A–D. Short-axis MR images of average quality obtained with conventional GRE (**A, B**) and multishot EPI (**C, D**) are shown at end-diastole (**A, C**) and end-systole (**B, D**). (Lamb et al. 1996). Note the typical breathing artifacts on the diastolic GRE image (**A**), such as signal voids in the anterolateral region of the LV and the fuzzy epicardial border at the posterior wall. Note differences in edge sharpness and contrast between blood and myocardium. For details concerning acquisition parameters see text. Practical details: The short-axis section levels are scanned separately during a single breath-hold in expiration with a maximal duration of 15 s. This procedure is repeated ten times to encompass the entire heart at ten section levels. The overall examination time, including breathing between the acquisitions, is approximately 7 min. This multishot, short-axis, breath-hold EPI technique for evaluating the heart provides accurate measurements of LV function and mass (Lamb et al. 1996). In addition to the shorter acquisition time of EPI its reduced image analysis time may contribute to a more widespread application of cardiac MRI. (From Lamb and de Roos 1996)

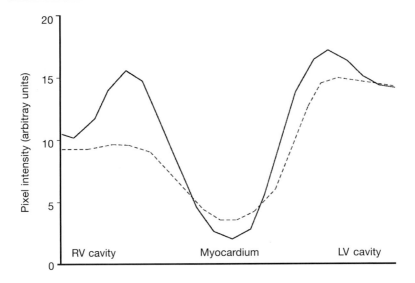

Fig. 16. Pixel intensity profiles along a line leading from the right ventricular (*RV*) cavity, across the septum (myocardium), to the left ventricular (*LV*) cavity on the end-diastolic images of Figure 15. Profiles were obtained from conventional GRE MRI (*dashed line*) and from EPI (*solid line*) displayed at the same window and level settings. Note differences in steepness and contrast between the profiles. (From Lamb et al. 1996)

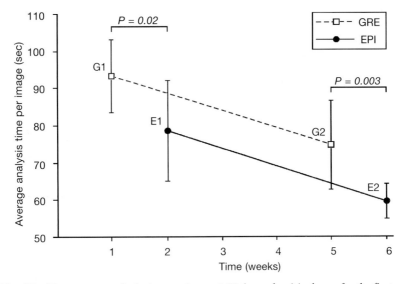

Fig. 17. The average analysis time per image ± SD (*error bars*) is shown for the first and second manual border tracings of the endocardium and epicardium on GRE- and EPI-derived images (G1, G2, E1, E2). Note the observed „learning effect" of an inexperienced observer. Differences between GRE and EPI and between the first and second reading were statistically significant ($p < 0.05$). (From Lamb et al. 1996)

3.3.2   Real-Time Respiratory Navigator Gating

Although the above described segmented EPI sequence is already being used routinely for evaluation of ischemic heart disease, variability in breath-hold levels may result in misregistration between imaging slice levels (Wang et al. 1995). Therefore alternatives for the breath-holding have been developed based on navigator echoes (Wang et al. 1996). Navigator echo signals can be acquired to sample the diaphragm position before and after the image data readout to gate the acquisition in real time (Figs. 18, 19; Wang et al. 1996). This technique also seems applicable to short-axis MRI of the heart.

Eliminating the need for breath-holds serves several clinically relevant purposes:

a) It obviates the need for breath-holding, thereby facilitating data acquisition, particularly under stress conditions.

b) Respiratory navigator gating allows averaging of multiple MR signals which by itself reduces motion artifacts and is ultimately suitable for imaging during cardiac stress.

c) It allows acquisition of images with a higher spatial resolution because more time is available for k-space sampling than during the 15 s breath-hold.

Initial results show that it is possible to obtain short-axis MR images of the LV using real-time respiratory navigator gating during continuous breathing with an image quality comparable to breath-hold acquisitions (Figs. 20, 21). This approach could substantially contribute to a more widespread application of cardiac functional MRI as well as for the morphological depiction of coronary arteries.

3.4   Myocardial Viability

The capability of gradient-echo MRI to provide functional information about the state of pathologically altered myocardium in combination with assessment of diastolic wall thickness and systolic wall thickening makes it suitable for identification of myocardial viability (Baer et al. 1994b, 1995). A comparison between wall thickness measurements by MRI with technetium-99m MIBI tomographic imaging showed an excellent correlation in patients with large chronic Q-wave infarcts. Baer et al. (1995) compared low-dose dobutamine MRI with positron emission tomography (PET) in 35 patients with myocardial infarction (> 4 months old). MRI was shown to be highly accurate in assessing myocardial viability. Viable myocardium was characterized by preserved end-diastolic wall thickness and a dobutamine-inducible contraction reserve, suggesting that both parameters should be taken into account to maximize the sensitivity of MRI for the detection of myocardial viability. Recovery of wall thickening under dobutamine stress appeared to be a better predictor of viability than PET. These findings are supported by Perrone-Filardi et al. (1992a,b) using PET with fluorine-18-fluorodeoxyglucose. In most regions with reduced end-diastolic wall thickness and absent wall thickening PET revealed the absence of metabolic activity, indicating the suitability of MRI in the assessment of myocardial viability.

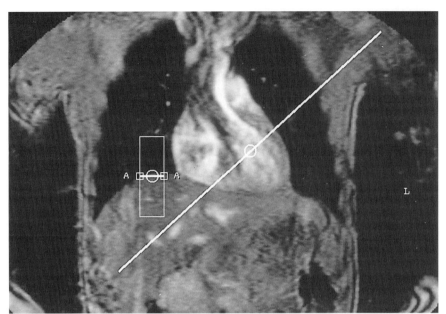

Fig. 18. A vertical navigator through the dome of the right hemidiaphragm is shown planned on a coronal survey image. The localized navigator echo consists of a spiral 25-mm diameter cylindrical excitation followed by a flow compensated readout along the long axis of the cylindrical excitation (McConnell et al. 1997). k-Space data from this readout are then Fourier transformed in real time, with the magnitude taken to give navigator image data (Fig. 19)

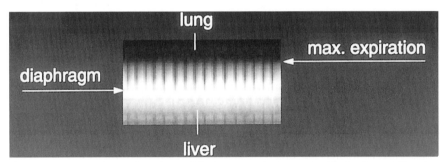

Fig. 19. Navigator image data obtained during 17 respiration cycles. The horizontal direction represents time, the vertical direction shows the oscillating displacement of the diaphragm level derived from the navigator beam. The navigator "position" was calculated prospectively for each heartbeat using a cross-correlation method. A user-selected portion ("kernel") of the navigator image data from a "reference" heartbeat was correlated to the navigator image data for each subsequent heartbeat. The kernel length of the reference image (80 mm) was chosen to include only the diaphragm and exclude relatively static tissues, such as the shoulders and chest wall. The navigator position measurement and analysis were performed in real time immediately before and after data collection (McConnell et al. 1997). Around expiration an acceptance "window" was specified which determines the maximum allowed respiratory excursion; k-space lines are then accepted for reconstruction of MR images. Usually this gating window ranges from 1 to 10 mm and depends on the specific breathing pattern of each subject. Resulting images are shown in Figure 20

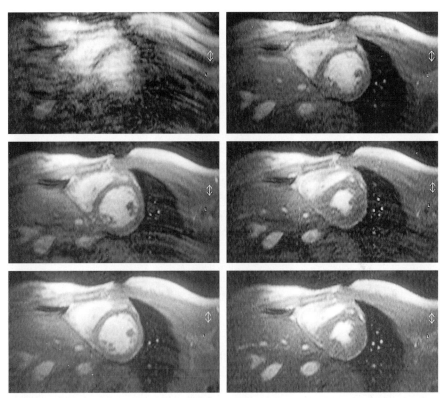

Fig. 20.   Short-axis views of the LV of a healthy volunteer. Images were acquired using a turbo-field-echo technique during continuous breathing (*upper left*), breath-holding (*upper right*), real-time respiratory navigator gating with a large acceptance window (10 mm, *middle images*), navigators with a smaller gating window (3 mm, *lower images*) both in end-diastole (*left*) and end-systole (*right*). Note the decrease in breathing artifacts when comparing the different gating window settings for the navigator acquisitions

Viability demonstrated by MRI as a contraction reserve in akinetic myocardium reveals the potential functional competence of the myocardium and may therefore be more predictive of recovery after revascularization than the detection of myocardial glycolytic activity by PET. PET may detect metabolic activity in myocardium with severe impairment of function with only small remnants of viable tissue, which do not show recovery of function during stress or after revascularization (Baer et al. 1995).

3.5   Stress MRI

Pharmacological stress has been applied during MRI for detection of functional abnormalities in patients with coronary artery disease because physical exercise during MRI is difficult to perform due to motion artifacts and space restriction.

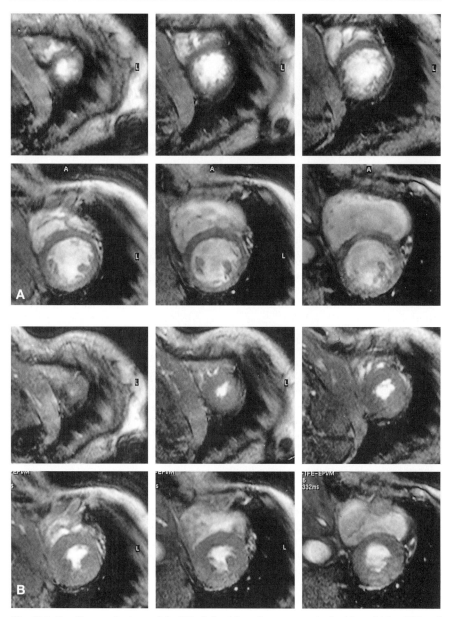

Fig. 21A, B.   Short-axis views of the LV of a healthy volunteer acquired with multishot EPI and real-time respiratory navigator gating during continuous breathing. Six slices of a dataset covering the entire LV are shown at end-diastole (**A**) and end-systole (**B**)

Dobutamine stress may be more reliable than dipyridamole stress for inducing wall motion abnormalities in patients with coronary artery disease, whereas dipyridamole stress should be reserved for myocardial perfusion imaging. Dobutamine is a synthetic catecholamine with relatively selective positive inotropic stimulation. The action begins within 2 min following administration and the maximal effect occurs after 10–14 min. Pharmacological stress using dobutamine has a number of advantages, including the ease of administration by a peripheral vein, the close resemblance to physical exercise, the short half-life of the drug, high tolerance, and safety and the extensive clinical experience with the agent. Dobutamine increases myocardial oxygen consumption by augmenting contractility and heart rate. Hence a marked imbalance between myocardial oxygen demand and supply may occur, resulting in myocardial ischemia.

Under dobutamine stress wall motion abnormalities may occur as an early manifestation of myocardial ischemia. The occurrence of ventricular arrhythmias is an infrequent but potentially serious side effect of dobutamine administration. Pennell et al. (1992) studied 22 patients with coronary artery disease both by dobutamine MRI and thallium tomography. Comparison of perfusion defects and wall motion abnormalities during stress showed 90% agreement, and dobutamine infusion was well-tolerated in all patients. Van Rugge et al. (1993a) identified wall motion dynamics in 23 healthy volunteers, and provided calculations of segmental wall thickening and hemodynamic parameters using dobutamine stress imaging. In 37 patients with coronary artery disease van Rugge et al. (1993b) showed an overall sensitivity of 81% and a specificity of 100% in detecting coronary artery disease when using dobutamine MRI; in patients with single-, double-, and triple-vessel disease the sensitivity values were 75%, 80%, and 100%, respectively. A subsequent study comprising 39 consecutive patients with clinically suspected coronary artery disease referred for coronary arteriography showed that dobutamine-stress MRI identifies wall motion abnormalities by quantitative analysis using the centerline method (van Rugge et al. 1994); the sensitivity, specificity, and accuracy were 91%, 80%, and 90%, respectively.

These findings were corroborated by Baer et al. (1994a), who studied 28 patients with dobutamine MRI and found an overall sensitivity of 87% and a specificity of 100% for the detection of coronary artery disease. In another study Baer et al. (1994b) compared the findings of dobutamine MRI with dobutamine-stress technetium-99m MIBI tomographic imaging in 35 patients with coronary artery disease; a high correlation between the two imaging modalities was found with respect to the detection of a dobutamine-induced ischemic response. These studies illustrate the feasibility of fast MR stress imaging strategies in the assessment of reversible myocardial ischemia.

3.6   Summary

Fast MR data acquisition techniques provide the basis for developing a comprehensive cardiac examination. Assessment of myocardial perfusion, wall motion, coronary flow reserve, and morphological depiction of coronary arteries have all been rendered within reach by the rapid technological developments in fast MRI. Much work remains to be carried out prior to a meaningful clinical implementation of these techniques in the routine assessment of patients with coronary artery disease.

References

Alfidi RJ, Masaryk TJ, Haacke EM, Lenz GW, Ross JS, Modic MT, Nelson AD, LiPuma JP, Cohen AM (1987) MR angiography of peripheral, carotid, and coronary arteries. AJR Am J Roentgenol 149:1097–1109

Atkinson D, Burstein D, Edelman RR (1990) First-pass cardiac perfusion: evaluation with ultrafast MR imaging. Radiology 174:757–762

Baer FM, Voth E, Theissen P, Schicha H, Sechtem U (1994a) Gradient-echo magnetic resonance imaging during incremental dobutamine infusion for the localization of coronary artery stenoses. Eur Heart J 15:218–225

Baer FM, Voth E, Theissen P, Schneider CA, Schicha H, Sechtem U (1994b) Coronary artery disease: findings with GRE MR imaging and Tc-99m-methoxyisobutyl-isonitrile SPECT during simultaneous dobutamine stress. Radiology 193:203–209

Baer FM, Voth E, Schneider CA, Theissen P, Schicha H, Sechtem U (1995) Comparison of low-dose dobutamine-gradient-echo magnetic resonance imaging and positron emission tomography with [18F]fluorodeoxyglucose in patients with chronic coronary artery disease. A functional and morphological approach to the detection of residual myocardial viability. Circulation 91:1006–1015

Baldy C, Douek P, Croisille P, Magnin IE, Revel D, Amiel M (1994) Automated myocardial edge detection from breath-hold cine-MR images: evaluation of left ventricular volume and mass. Magn Reson Imag 12:589–598

Butts K, Riederer SJ, Ehman RL, Felmlee JP, Grimm RC (1993) Echo-planar imaging of the liver with a standard MR imaging system. Radiology 189:259–264

Butts K, Riederer SJ, Ehman RL, Thompson RM, Jack CR (1994) Interleaved echo planar imaging on a standard MRI system. Magn Reson Med 31:67–72

Cho ZH, Mun CW, Friedenberg RM (1991) NMR angiography of coronary vessels with 2-D planar image scanning. Magn Reson Med 20:134–143

Constable RT, Rath KM, Sinusas AJ, Gore JC (1994) Development and evaluation of tracking algorithms for cardiac wall motion analysis using phase velocity MR imaging. Magn Reson Med 32:33–42

Davis CP, McKinnon GC, Debatin JF, Wetter D, Eichenberger AC, Duewell S, Von Schulthess GK (1994) Normal heart: evaluation with echo-planar MR imaging. Radiology 191:691–696

Davis CP, McKinnon GC, Debatin JF, Duewell S, von Schulthess GK (1995) Single-shot versus interleaved echo-planar MR imaging: application to visualization of cardiac valve leaflets. J Magn Reson Imaging 5:107–112

Davis CP, Liu PF, Hauser M, Gohde SC, Von Schulthess GK, Debatin JF (1997) Coronary flow and coronary flow reserve measurements in humans with breath held magnetic resonance phase contrast velocity mapping. Magn Reson Med 37:537–544

de Roos A, van Rossum AC, van der Wall EE (1989) Reperfused and nonreperfused myocardial infarction: potential of gadolinium-DTPA enhanced MR imaging. Radiology 172:717–720

de Roos A, Matheijssen NAA, Doornbos J, van Dijkman PRM, van Voorthuisen AE, van der Wall EE (1990) Myocardial infarct size after reperfusion therapy: assessment with Gd-DTPA-enhanced MR imaging. Radiology 176:517–521

Dendale P, Franken P, Meusel M, van der Geest R, de Roos A (1997) Distinction between open and occluded and infarct-related arteries using contrast-enhanced magnetic resonance imaging. Am J Cardiol 80:334–336

Doorey AJ, Wills JS, Blasetto J, Goldenberg EM (1994) Usefulness of magnetic resonance imaging for diagnosing an anomalous coronary artery coursing between aorta and pulmonary trunk. Am J Cardiol 74:198–199

Doyle M, Scheidegger MB, de Graaf RG, Vermeulen J, Pohost GM (1993) Coronary artery imaging in multiple 1-sec breath holds. Magn Reson Imaging 11:3–6

Duerinckx AJ, Bogaert J, Jiang H, Lewis BS (1995) Anomalous origin of the left coronary artery: diagnosis by coronary MR angiography. AJR Am J Roentgenol 164:1095–1097

Edelman RR, Wallner B, Singer A, Atkinson DJ, Saini S (1990) Segmented turboFLASH: method for breath-hold MR imaging of the liver with flexible contrast. Radiology 177:515–521

Edelman RR, Manning WJ, Burstein D, Paulin S (1991) Coronary arteries: breath-hold MR angiography. Radiology 181:641–643

Edelman RR, Wielopolski P, Schmitt F (1994) Echo-planar MR imaging. Radiology 192:600–612

Eichenberger AC, Schuiki E, Kochli VD, Amann FW, McKinnon GC, von Schulthess GK (1994) Ischemic heart disease: assessment with gadolinium-enhanced ultrafast MR imaging and dipyridamole stress (see comments) J Magn Reson Imaging 4:425–431

Eichstaedt HW, Felix R, Dougherty FC, Langer M, Rutsch W, Schmutzler H (1986) Magnetic resonance imaging in different stages of myocardial infarction using the contrast agent gadolinium-DTPA. Clin Cardiol 9:527–535

Fischer SE, Groen JP, Henson RE, White CA, Watkins MP, Wickline SA, Lorenz CH (1997) Myocardial perfusion assessment of the entire heart. Conf. Proc, Int Soc Magn Reson Med, p. 2065

Furber A, Lethimonnier F, Geslin P, L'hoste P, Suminski M, Tadei A, Jallet P, Caron-Poitreau C, Lejeune JJ (1997) Flow velocity quantitation in coronary arteries. Comparison between intravascular Doppler US and breath-hold MR angiograpy. Conf. Proc, Int Soc Magn Reson Med, p. 445

Globits S, Sakuma H, Shimakawa A, Foo TKF, Higgins CB (1997) Measurement of coronary blood flow velocity during handgrip exercise using breath hold velocity encoded cine magnetic resonance imaging. Am J Cardiol 79:234–237

Grist TM, Polzin JA, Bianco JA, Foo TKF, Bernstein MA, Mistretta CM (1997) Measurement of coronary blood flow and flow reserve using magnetic resonance imaging. Cardiology 88:80–89

Heid O (1997) True FISP cardiac fluoroscopy. Conf. Proc, Int Soc Magn Reson Med, p. 320

Hennig J, Schneider B (1997) Analysis of myocardial motion based on velocity measurements with a black-blood prepared segmented gradient echo sequence: methodology and applications to normal volunteers and patients. J Magn Reson Imaging (submitted)

Higgins CB, Saeed M, Wendland M, Yu K, Lauerma K, Dulce M, Kanth N (1993) Contrast media for cardiothoracic MR imaging. J Magn Reson Imaging 3:265–276

Holman ER, Buller VGM, de Roos A, van der Geest RJ, Baur LHB, van der Laarse A, Bruschke AVG, Reiber JHC, van der Wall EE (1997) Detection and quantification of dysfunctional myocardium by magnetic resonance imaging: a new three dimensional method for quantitative wall thickening analysis. Circulation 95:924–931

Hunter GJ, Hamberg LM, Weisskoff RM, Halpern EF, Brady TJ (1994) Measurement of stroke volume and cardiac output within a single breath hold with echo-planar MR imaging. J Magn Reson Imaging 4:51–58

Jerosch-Herold M, Wilke N, Wang Y, Stillman AE (1997) Can absolute myocardial bloodflow be quantified with the MR first pass technique and an extracellular contrast agent? Conf. Proc, Int Soc Magn Reson Med, p. 841

Johns JA, Leavitt MB, Newell JB (1990) Quantitation of acute myocardial infarct size by nuclear magnetic resonance imaging. J Am Coll Cardiol 15:143–149

Johnston DL, Mulvagh SL, Cashion RW, O'Neill PG, Roberts R, Rokey R (1989) Nuclear magnetic resonance imaging of acute myocardial infarction within 24 hours of chest pain onset. Am J Cardiol 64:172–176

Keijer JT, van Rossum AC, van Eenige MJ, Karreman AJ, Hofman MB, Valk J, Visser CA (1995) Semiquantitation of regional myocardial blood flow in normal human subjects by first-pass magnetic resonance imaging. Am Heart J 130:893–901

Kerr A, Pauly J, Hu B, Li K, Hardy C, Meyer C, Macovski A, Nishimura D (1997) Real-time interactive MRI on a conventional scanner. Conf. Proc, Int Soc Magn Reson Med, p. 319

Kim RJ, Lima JAC, Chen EL, Reeder SB, Klock FJ, Zerhouni EA, Judd RM (1997) Fast na 23 magnetic resonance imaging of acute reperfused myocardial infarction: potential to assess myocardial viability. Circulation 95:1877–1885

Kramer CM, Geskin G, Rogers WJ, Theobald TM, Hu Y-L, Reichek N (1997) Assessment of myocardial viability after reperfused first infarction by low dose dobutamine MR tagging. Conf. Proc, Int Soc Magn Reson Med, p. 387

Lamb HJ, de Roos A (1996) MRI in ischemic heart disease. Internet: http://medic-online.net/mr/deroos

Lamb HJ, Doornbos J, van der Velde EA, Kruit MC, Reiber JH, de Roos A (1996) Echo planar MRI of the heart on a standard system: validation of measurements of left ventricular function and mass. J Comput Assist Tomogr 20:942–949

Lotan CS, Cranney GB, Bouchard A, Bittner V, Prohost GM (1989) The value of cine nuclear magnetic resonance imaging for assessing regional ventricular function. J Am Coll Cardiol 14:1721–1729

Manning WJ, Atkinson DJ, Grossman W, Paulin S, Edelman RR (1991) First-pass nuclear magnetic resonance imaging studies using gadolinium-DTPA in patients with coronary artery disease. J Am Coll Cardiol 18:959–965

Manning WJ, Li W, Boyle NG, Edelman RR (1993a) Fat-suppressed breath-hold magnetic resonance coronary angiography. Circulation 87:94–104

Manning WJ, Li W, Edelman RR (1993b) A preliminary report comparing magnetic resonance coronary angiography with conventional angiography (comments). N Engl J Med 328:828–832 (erratum 330:152)

Mansfield P (1977) Multi-planar image formation using NMR spin echoes. J Phys C10:L55–L58

Matheijssen NAA, De Roos A, van der Wall EE, Doornbos J, van Dijkman PRM, Bruschke AVG, van Voorthuisen AE (1991) Acute myocardial infarction: comparison of T2-weighted and T1-weighted gadolinium-DTPA enhanced MR imaging. Magn Reson Med 17:460–469

Matheijssen NAA, Louwerenburg HW, van Rugge FP, Arens RPJH, Kauer B, de Roos A, van der Wall EE (1996) Comparison of ultrafast dipyridamole magnetic resonance imaging with dipyridemole sestaMIBI SPECT for detection of perfusion abnormalities in patients with one-vessel coronary artery disease: assessment by quantitative model fitting. Magn Reson Med 35:221–228

McConnell MV, Khasgiwala VC, Savord BJ, Chen MH, Chuang ML, Edelman RR, Manning WJ (1997) Prospective adaptive navigator correction for breath-hold MR coronary angiography. Magn Reson Med 37:148–152

McKinnon GC (1993) Ultrafast interleaved gradient-echo-planar imaging on a standard scanner. Magn Reson Med 30:609–616

McVeigh ER (1996) MRI of myocardial function: motion tracking techniques. Magn Reson Imaging 14:137–150

Meyer CH, Hu BS, Kerr AB, Sachs TS, Pauly JM, Macovski A, Nishimure DG (1997) High-resolution multislice spiral coronary angiography with real-time interactive localization. Conf. Proc, Int Soc Magn Reson Med, p. 439

Meyer CH, Hu BS, Nishimura DG, Macovski A (1992) Fast spiral coronary artery imaging. Magn Reson Med 28:202–213

Nishimura T, Kobayashi H, Ohara Y (1989a) Serial assessment of myocardial infarction by using gated MR imaging and Gd-DTPA. AJR Am J Roentgenol 153:715–720

Nishimura T, Yamada Y, Hayashi M (1989b) Determination of infarct size of acute myocardial infarction in dogs by magnetic resonance imaging and Gadolinium-DTPA: comparison with indium-111 antimyosin imaging. Am J Physiol Imaging 4:83–88

Oshinski JN, Hofland L, Mukundan S, Dixon WT, Parks WJ, Pettigrew RI (1996) Two dimensional coronary mr angiography without breath holding. Radiology 201:737–743

Pattynama PMT, Lamb HJL, van der Velde EA, van der Wall EE, De Roos A (1993) Left ventricular measurements with cine and spin-echo MR imaging: a study of reproducibility with variance component analysis. Radiology 187:261–268

Paulin S, Von Schulthess G, Fossel E, Krayenbuehl HP (1987) MR imaging of the aortic root and proximal coronary arteries. AJR Am J Roentgenol 148:665–670

Pelc LR, Sayre J, Yun K, Castro LJ, Herfkens RJ, Miller DC, Pelc NJ (1994) Evaluation of myocardial motion tracking with cine-phase contrast magnetic resonance imaging. Invest Radiol 29:1038–1042

Pennell DJ, Underwood SR, Ell PJ, Swanton RH, Walker JM, Longmore DB (1990a) Dipyridamole magnetic resonance imaging: a comparison with thallium-201 emission tomography. Br Heart J 64:362–369

Pennell DJ, Underwood SR, Longmore DB (1990b) Detection of coronary artery disease using MR imaging with dipyridamole infusion. J Comput Assist Tomogr 14:167–170

Pennell DJ, Underwood SR, Manzara CC, Swanton RH, Walker JM, Ell PJ, Longmore DB (1992) Magnetic resonance imaging during dobutamine stress in coronary artery disease. Am J Cardiol 70:34–40

Pennell DJ, Keegan J, Firmin DN, Gatehouse PD, Underwood SR, Longmore DB (1993) Magnetic resonance imaging of coronary arteries: technique and preliminary results. Br Heart J 70:315–326

Perrone-Filardi P, Bacharach SL, Dilsizian V, Maurea S, Frank JA, Bonow RO (1992a) Regional left ventricular wall thickening. Relation to regional uptake of 18fluorodeoxyglucose and 201Tl in patients with chronic coronary artery disease and left ventricular dysfunction. Circulation 86:1125–1137

Perrone-Filardi P, Bacharach SL, Dilsizian V, Maurea S, Marin-Neto JA, Arrighi JA, Frank JA, Bonow RO (1992b) Metabolic evidence of viable myocardium in regions with reduced wall thickness and absent wall thickening in patients with chronic ischemic left ventricular dysfunction. J Am Coll Cardiol 20:161–168

Pflugfelder PW, Sechtem UP, White RD, Higgins CB (1988) Quantification of regional myocardial function by rapid cine MR imaging. AJR Am J Roentgenol 150:523–529

Poncelet BP, Weisskoff RM, Wedeen VJ, Brady TJ, Kantor H (1993) Time of flight quantification of coronary flow with echo-planar MRI. Magn Reson Med 30:447–457

Post JC, van Rossum AC, Bronzwaer JG, de Cock CC, Hofman MB, Valk J, Visser CA (1995) Magnetic resonance angiography of anomalous coronary arteries. A new gold standard for delineating the proximal course? Circulation 92:3163–3171

Post JC, van Rossum AC, Hofman MB, Valk J, Visser CA (1996) Three-dimensional respiratory-gated MR angiography of coronary arteries: comparison with conventional coronary angiography. AJR Am J Roentgenol 166:1399–1404

Rzedzian RR, Pykett IL (1987) Instant images of the human heart using a new, whole-body MR imaging system. AJR Am J Roentgenol 149:245–250

Sakuma H, Blake LM, Amidon TM, O'Sullivan M, Szolar DH, Furber AP, Bernstein MA, Foo TK, Higgins CB (1996) Coronary flow reserve: noninvasive measurement in humans with breath-hold velocity-encoded cine MR imaging. Radiology 198:745–750

Sakuma H, Fujita N, Foo TKF, Caputo GR, Nelson SJ, Hartiala J, Shimakawa A, Higgins CB (1993) Evaluation of left ventricular volume and mass with breath-hold cine MR imaging. Radiology 188:377–380

Sechtem U, Pflugfelder P, Higgins CB (1987) Quantification of cardiac function by conventional and cine magnetic resonance imaging. Cardiovasc Intervent Radiol 10:365–373

Stehling M, Chapman B, Glover P, Ordidge RJ, Mansfield P, Dutka D, Howseman A, Coxon R, Turner R, Jaroszkiewicz G, Morris GK, Worthington BS, Coupland RE (1987) Real-time NMR imaging of coronary vessels. Lancet II:964–965

Stuber M, Scheidegger MB, Boesiger P (1997) Realtime imaging of the heart. Conf. Proc, Int Soc Magn Reson Med, p. 908

Szolar DH, Saeed M, Wendland MF, Sakuma H, Roberts TPL, Stiskal MA, Derugin N, Higgins CB (1996) MR imaging characterization of postischemic myocardial dysfunction (stunned myocardium): relationship between functional and perfusion abnormalities. J Magn Reson Imaging 6:615–624

Unterweger M, Debatin JF, Leung DA, Wildermuth S, McKinnon GC, Vonschulthess GK (1994) Cardiac volumetry: comparison of echoplanar and conventional cine magnetic resonance data acquisition strategies. Invest Radiol 29:994–1000

van der Wall EE, Vliegen HW, de Roos A, Bruschke AV (1995) Magnetic resonance imaging in coronary artery disease. Circulation 92:2723–2739

van Dijkman PRM, van der Wall EE, De Roos A, Matheijssen NAA, van Rossum AC, Doornbos J, van der Laarse A, van Voorthuisen AE, Bruschke AVG (1991) Acute, subacute and chronic myocardial infarction: quantitative analysis of gadolinium-enhanced MR images. Radiology 180:147–151

van Rossum AC, Visser FC, van Eenige MJ (1990) Value of gadolinium-diethylenetriaminepentaacetic acid dynamics in magnetic resonance imaging of acute myocardial infarction with occluded and reperfused coronary arteries after thrombolysis. Am J Cardiol 65:845–851

van Rugge FP, Boreel JJ, van der Wall EE, van Dijkman PRM, van der Laarse A, Doornbos J, De Roos A, Den Boer JA, Bruschke AVG, van Voorthuisen AE (1991) Cardiac first-pass and myocardial perfusion in normal subjects assessed by subsecond Gd-DTPA enhanced MR imaging. J Comput Assist Tomogr 15:959–965

van Rugge F, van der Wall E, van Dijkman P, Louwerenburg H, de Roos A, Bruschke A (1992a) Usefulness of ultrafast magnetic resonance imaging in healed myocardial infarction. Am J Cardiol 70:1233–1237

van Rugge FP, van der Wall EE, Bruschke AVG (1992b) New developments in pharmacologic stress imaging. Am Heart J 124:468–485

van Rugge FP, Holman ER, van der Wall EE, de Roos A, van der Laarse A, Bruschke AVG (1993a) Quantitation of global and regional left ventricular function by cine magnetic resonance imaging during dobutamine stress in normal human subjects. Eur Heart J 14:456–463 van Rugge FP, van der Wall EE, de Roos A, Bruschke AV (1993b) Dobutamine stress magnetic resonance imaging for detection of coronary artery disease. J Am Coll Cardiol 22:431–439

van Rugge FP, van der Wall EE, Spanjersberg SJ, de Roos A, Matheijssen NA, Zwinderman AH, van Dijkman PR, Reiber JH, Bruschke AV (1994) Magnetic resonance imaging during dobutamine stress for detection and localization of coronary artery disease. Quantitative wall motion analysis using a modification of the centerline method. Circulation 90:127–138

Vliegen HW, Doornbos J, Deroos A, Jukema JW, Bekedam MA, Vanderwall EE (1997) Value of fast gradient echo magnetic resonance angiography as an adjunct to coronary arteriography in detecting and confirming the course of clinically significant coronary artery anomalies. Am J Cardiol 79:773–776

Wang SJ, Hu BS, Macovski A, Nishimura DG (1991) Coronary angiography using fast selective inversion recovery. Magn Reson Med 18:417–423

Wang Y, Riederer SJ, Ehman RL (1995) Respiratory motion of the heart: kinematics and the implications for the spatial resolution in coronary imaging. Magn Reson Imag 33:713–719

Wang Y, Rossman PJ, Grimm RC, Riederer SJ, Ehman RL (1996) Navigator-echo-based real-time respiratory gating and triggering for reduction of respiration effects in three-dimensional coronary MR angiography. Radiology 198:55–60

Wedeen VJ (1992) Magnetic resonance imaging of myocardial kinematics. Technique to detect, localize, and quantify the strain rates of the active human myocardium. Magn Reson Med 27:52–67

Wetter DR, McKinnon GC, Debatin JF, von Schulthess GK (1995) Cardiac echo-planar MR imaging: Comparison of single- and multi-shot techniques. Radiology 194:765–770

Wilke N, Simm C, Zhang J, Ellermann J, Ya X, Merkle H, Path G, Ludemann H, Bache RJ, Ugurbil K (1993) Contrast-enhanced first pass myocardial perfusion imaging: correlation between myocardial blood flow in dogs at rest and during hyperemia. Magn Reson Med 29:485–497

Wisenberg G, Finnie KJ, Jablonsky G, Kostuk WJ, Marshall T (1988) Nuclear magnetic resonance and radionuclide angiographic assessment of acute myocardial infarction in a randomized of intravenous streptokinase. Am J Cardiol 62:1011–1016

Wood AM, Hoffmann KR, Lipton MJ (1994) Cardiac function: quantification with magnetic resonance and computed tomography. Radiol Clin North Am 32:553–579

Yang P, Kerr A, Liu A, Pauly J, Hardy C, Meyer C, Macovski A, Hu B (1997) Real-time interactive cardiac MRI for patients with suboptimal echocardiographic studies. Conf. Proc, Int Soc Magn Reson Med, p. 909

4   Ultrafast Magnetic Resonance Imaging of the Vascular System

D.A. LEUNG and J.F. DEBATIN

1   Introduction

Motion sensitivity inherent to the magnetic resonance (MR) experiment has been exploited for noninvasive vascular imaging since the early days of MR imaging (MRI). Based on the effect of blood flow onto the signal amplitude and phase, time-of-flight (TOF) and phase-contrast (PC) MR angiography (MRA) techniques were developed. Both forms of MRA are totally noninvasive, not associated with any known side effects, and can easily be performed as an outpatient examination, eliminating the need for costly postprocedure patient monitoring. Lengthy data acquisition times, image degrading artifacts due to both voluntary and involuntary (respiratory and cardiac) motion, and in-plane dephasing, combined with limited signal-to-noise (SNR) and spatial resolution have limited the integration of these conventional MRA techniques into meaningful clinical routines outside the cerebrum.

The implementation of stronger and faster gradient systems has laid the foundation for vast reductions in MR data acquisition times. Complex 3D gradient echo data sets can now be collected within a single breath-hold, virtually eliminating respiration induced adverse effects on image quality. In analogy to computed tomographic (CT) angiography, the MR data acquisition speed has become sufficiently fast to exploit the arterial phase of intravenously administered contrast agents. In combination, these factors have provided the basis for ultrafast T1-weighted contrast-enhanced 3D MRA. Not based on flow effects but on the T1-shortening effects of paramagnetic contrast within the vessels under consideration, this technique overcomes most of the limitations inherent to conventional MRA. The technique's striking success is reflected by its rapid integration into routine clinical imaging protocols in centers throughout the world. Thus contrast-enhanced 3D MRA is being increasingly accepted as a credible noninvasive alternative to conventional catheter angiography for assessing the arterial system in the chest, abdomen, pelvis, and periphery.

In addition to accelerating conventional gradient echo sequences, echo-planar imaging (EPI), as first described by Mansfield in 1977, now also appears practical. Although echo-planar techniques have not gained entry into routine clinical imaging protocols, they do provide an interesting potential means to improve the morphological and functional MR-based evaluation of vascular structures. The application of echo-planar data-acquisition strategies to MRA reduces data-acquisition times sharply, enabling the breath-held acquisition of data covering an entire vascular territory. Furthermore, cardiac motion can be resolved by acquiring data only during certain portions of the cardiac cycle. Finally, echo-planar MRA may take advantage of short-lived performance-enhancing measures, such as arterial and venous flow augmentation.

In addition to the morphological assessment of vascular disease, MRI offers the possibility of obtaining functional information capable of mapping blood flow velocities and volumes over time. Here too the integration of ultrafast data acquisition strategies has enhanced the technique's applicability. Measurement accuracy has been enhanced in two ways:

a) by enabling breath-held data acquisition the corrupting influence of respiratory motion has been eliminated, and

b) by permitting better temporal resolution the effects of temporal averaging have been mitigated.

This review explores the opportunities presented by fast and ultrafast MR data-acquisition strategies regarding the morphological and functional assessment of the vascular system.

2   Vascular Morphology

Ultrafast MRA techniques allowing data acquisition in apnea have considerably extended the clinical utility of MRA to encompass the vasculature subject to respiratory motion in the abdomen and thorax. Technical aspects and clinical applications of contrast-enhanced 3D MRA and echo-planar MRA are discussed in the following sections.

2.1   Contrast-Enhanced 3D MRA

2.1.1   Technical Aspects

Contrast-enhanced 3D MRA fundamentally differs from other vascular MRI strategies in that it is not flow dependent. Blood signal is derived from the T_1-shortening effect of the dynamically infused paramagnetic contrast agent. Hence arterial contrast is based on the difference in T_1 relaxation between blood and surrounding tissue. As a result saturation problems associated with slow flow and turbulence-induced signal voids are overcome. Large 3D volumes can be acquired with the imaging plane oriented along the long-axis of the vessels of interest.

2.1.1.1 Hardware Considerations

3D contrast-enhanced MRA can essentially be performed on any MR system. The gradient strength of a given system determines the time required for data acquisition. In its initial implementation for aortoiliac inflow assessment using conventional gradients, imaging times ranged from 3 to 5 min, depending on the number of sections acquired (Prince et al. 1993). The 3D data were collected during shallow respiration. Although image quality was sufficient for visualization of large vessels, it was recognized that smaller vessels, particularly those subject to respiratory motion, such as the distal renal arteries, were not adequately resolved for diagnostic purposes. Similar observations have been made with 3D gadolinium MRA of the thorax (Prince et al. 1996).

High-performance gradient systems allow a reduction in imaging times such that an entire 3D data set can be sampled within a comfortable breath-hold interval. Images thus obtained have been shown to significantly improve image quality (Prince et al. 1995a; Leung et al. 1996). Short acquisition times are achieved by a considerable reduction in the repetition time (TR). Gradient switching capabilities with an achievable slew rate in the region of 100–120 mT m^{-1} ms^{-1} should be considered a prerequisite for breath-hold gadolinium MRA. Such hardware is commercially available and implemented in a growing number of MR systems.

As with conventional MRI, better image quality can be expected with the use of a phased-array surface coil for signal reception.

2.1.1.2 Pulse Sequence

The pulse sequence generally used for contrast-enhanced MRA is a fast 3D Fourier transform gradient-recalled echo (GRE) sequence. T1-weighting combined with background suppression is ensured by spoiling, which can be accomplished by radio frequency or gradient techniques. With high-performance gradient systems the TR should be reduced to approximately 3–7 ms and the echo time (TE) to about 1–3 ms (Prince et al. 1995a,b). Future improvements in gradient switching capabilities will likely further reduce the minimum TR and TE achievable. Several other parameters play a role in minimizing the imaging time. A rather high sampling bandwidth setting needs to be used, albeit at the cost of a slight relative reduction in SNR. The spatial resolution can be maximized within the limits of the breath-hold capabilities of a given patient by adjusting the matrix size and number of slices and the use af a rectangular field of view (FOV). Finally, partial Fourier methods (otherwise known as fractional NEX) can be employed, which considerably shorten acquisition times. A flip angle of 30°–50° has been shown to provide optimal results (Prince 1994; Prince et al. 1995a,b). Further reductions in TR may warrant use of a smaller flip angle to ensure sufficient arterial signal.

It is advisable to obtain a precontrast data set in order to check correct placement of the imaging volume and for the patient to practice maintaining a breath-hold during the entire data acquisition period.

2.1.1.3 Gadolinium Infusion

Crucial to the quality of breath-hold contrast-enhanced 3D MRA images is the well-timed intravenous administration of paramagnetic contrast. An extracellular paramagnetic MR contrast agent such as a gadolinium chelate is infused via a peripheral venous access. The great advantage of these contrast agents is that they have no clinically detectable nephrotoxicity and can therefore be used in patients with renal insufficiency (Niendorf et al. 1991). In general, 0.2–0.3 mmol/kg body weight of the agent is administered. Current regulatory guidelines suggest a maximum dose of 0.3 mmol/kg although some centers have used a dosage up to 0.5 mmol/kg. A dose of 0.2 mmol/kg body weight has been shown to be optimal for most vascular territories (Hany et al., 1997c). The use of new contrast agents with increased T1 relaxivity, currently undergoing clinical testing, promises to reduce the dose requirements for contrast-enhanced MRA. Intravascular agents will allow acquisition of high resolution 3D data sets since the acquisition time is no longer limited to the arterial contrast phase. Such agents are currently under clinical evaluation.

Use of an automated infusion pump facilitates the contrast administration process. Hand injection from within the scanner room is feasible though slightly less reliable. Timing of the contrast application must be adjusted to ensure the presence of a high concentration of contrast material within the vessels of interest during acquisition of the central portion of k-space, responsible for the contrast-defining low spatial frequency image information. This corresponds to the midportion of the acquisition in conventionally encoded sequences. Poor timing of the contrast bolus results in insufficient signal within the vessel of interest if the bolus arrives too late, and venous/background overlap if bolus arrival occurs too early.

Estimates of contrast travel time from the venous access to the imaging volume should be sufficiently accurate to avoid nondiagnostic exams. Since the circulation time is difficult to predict based on available parameters such as age, body weight, or heart rate, the scan delay must be determined individually. For this purpose, a bolus-timing acquisition is performed prior to the acquisition of the 3D MRA data set (Hany et al. 1997a,b). Following the intravenous test bolus injection of 2–4 ml gadolinium, GRE images (multiphase) are acquired at fixed time intervals (every 1–2 s) through the vessels of interest for approximately 40 s. The bolus appearance time can be determined based on sequential signal intensity measurements in a region-of-interest placed within the vessel of interest. In this manner image acquisition can be timed such that the peak contrast concentration coincides with the sampling of the central orders of k-space.

2.1.1.4 Image Interpretation

Contrast-enhanced 3D MRA images are best interpreted on an independent workstation with 3D reconstruction capabilities. In addition to perusal of the original sections, diagnoses should be based on a combination of maximum intensity projection (MIP) images and interactive 3D multiplaner reformations (MPR) (Hany et al., 1997d). Surface rendering algorithms and subvolume MIP reconstructions are useful mainly for demonstration purposes. The MPR technique permits cross-sectional visualization of the vessels in any plane. Venous overlap can effectively be compensated for and the course of tortuous vessels can easily be reconstructed. This represents an advantage even over conventional catheter angiography.

2.1.2   Clinical Applications

2.1.2.1 Pulmonary Arteries

MRI of the pulmonary vasculature has been severely handicapped by respiratory and cardiac motion artifacts as well as by limited spatial resolution (Wielopolski et al. 1992; Foo et al. 1992). Although several studies have demonstrated reasonable diagnostic accuracy for the assessment of the central pulmonary arteries with conventional MRA techniques, the MR-based evaluation of patients with suspected pulmonary embolism has remained largely experimental. To date no conventional MRA technique has been able to match the advances in CT angiography for the diagnosis of central and paracentral pulmonary embolism. On GRE images a thrombus generally appears as a "filling defect." However, in patients with slow blood flow it is often difficult to differentiate between thrombus and signal void or inhomogeneity caused by saturation effects.

Contrast-enhanced 3D MRA provides homogeneous intravascular signal independent of flow velocity (Fig. 1). Hence a thrombus appears as a true filling defect (Fig. 2). The large 3D volume allows evaluation of the entire pulmonary vasculature with sufficient spatial resolution. Initial experience with breath-hold

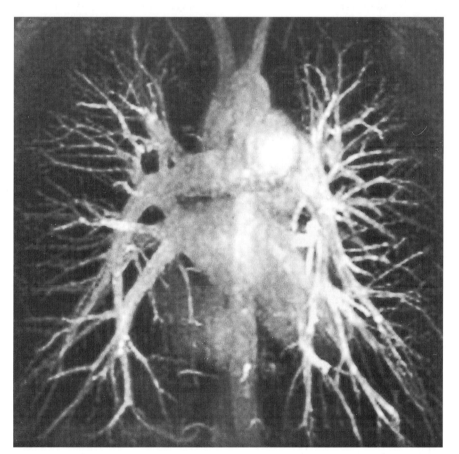

Fig. 1. MIP display of a 3D gadolinium MR pulmonary angiogram of a normal volunteer acquired during a breath-hold interval of 27 s. Note depiction of pulmonary arteries to the subsegmental level

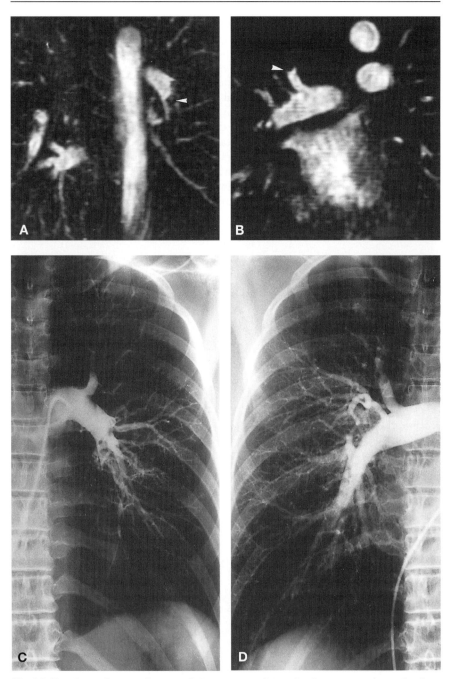

Fig. 2A–D. Coronal source images of 3D contrast-enhanced pulmonary angiography show embolic occlusion of the left interlobar artery (**A**, *arrowhead*) and the right upper lobe artery (**B**, *arrowhead*). Analogous findings in the conventional pulmonary angiogram (**C, D**)

contrast-enhanced 3D MRA in a group of volunteers showed that the pulmonary arteries can be evaluated to the segmental and subsegmental levels in 100% and 81%, respectively (Steiner et al. 1997). In a series of 30 patients, the 3D technique demonstrated sensitivities ranging from 75% to 100% and specificities ranging from 95% to 100% for the detection of pulmonary embolism, as compared with conventional angiography (Meaney et al. 1997b). Since venous overlap is almost unavoidable in pulmonary artery imaging, it is particularly important to base the ultimate diagnosis on multiplanar reformations.

For diagnostic images it must be considered crucial to acquire the data during a breath-hold interval of reasonably short duration. Most patients with suspected pulmonary embolism are severely dyspnoic and do not tolerate apnea exceeding 15 s. In patients who cannot hold their breath for even that long the acquisition can be shortened by reducing the spatial resolution or the number of acquired sections.

2.1.2.2 Aorta

Aortic Dissection.   Beyond establishing the presence of dissection, it is crucial to define the localization and extent of disease. Owing to the severe therapeutic consequences the diagnostic test employed must possess high sensitivity and specificity. Breath-held contrast-enhanced 3D MRA can help meet these diagnostic requirements. The technique is fast and combines the advantages of arterial contrast, similar to conventional contrast angiography, with cross-sectional information. Since image quality is not affected by slow flow, differentiation of thrombus from slow flow is always possible (Fig. 3). Using MPR, it is possible to locate the site of intimal perforation and aortic branch vessel involvement in most cases (Fig. 4). In a recent study assessing 90 patients with conventional angiographic or surgical correlation, nonbreath-hold contrast-enhanced 3D MRA correctly diagnosed the type of aortic dissection in 100% (Prince et al. 1996). In addition, patency of the false lumen and entry and reentry tears were identified in all cases. Regarding the analysis of aortic branch vessel involvement, breath-holding has been shown to be of eminent importance.

Aortic Aneurysm.   In addition to establishing the presence and extent of aneurysmal changes, a diagnostic test should also assess for periaortic hematoma and associated stenoses of branch vessels. Conventional MRA techniques do not reliably detect accessory renal arteries or depict associated occlusive disease of aortic branch vessels and pelvic arteries. Moreover, slow flow within aneurysms and turbulent flow in stenoses can make identification of thrombosis and grading of stenoses problematic. Helical CT has shown potential for the evaluation of aortic branches if narrow collimation is used (Galanski et al. 1993). Unfortunately this limits the FOV obtainable to only a portion of the abdominal aorta (Rubin et al. 1994). Breath-held, contrast-enhanced 3D MRA improves MR examinations by providing exact topographic information on the aneurysmal lumen and its relationship to aortic branch vessels (Fig. 5). Recent studies comparing contrast-enhanced 3D MRA with conventional angiography and operative findings of abdominal aortic aneurysms demonstrated high sensitivity and

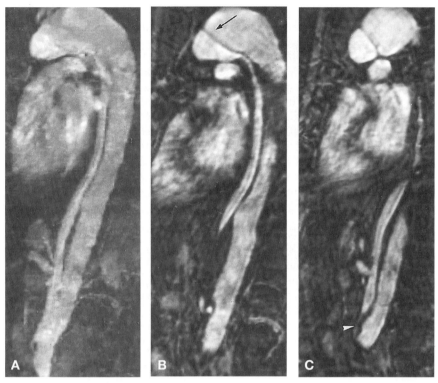

Fig. 3A–C. A 45-year-old patient with type B dissection. MIP of contrast-enhanced 3D MRA (**A**) demonstrating the extent of the dissection. Note enhancement of both true and false channels. Sagittal 3D reformations (**B, C**) showing the entry (*arrow*) and reentry (*arrowhead*) tears

specificity for detecting occlusive lesions of splanchnic, renal and iliac arteries, as well as accessory renal arteries (Prince et al. 1995a,b; Kaufmann et al. 1994). Important preoperative information regarding associated disease of the renal arteries and their relationship to the proximal neck of the aneurysm can easily be obtained from multiplanar reformations (Fig. 5). To permit analysis of the abdominal aortic wall and facilitate the delineation of thrombosed regions, it is useful to acquire a T1-weighted sequence postcontrast (Fig. 6). Enhancement of the aortic wall is indicative of an inflammatory aneurysm.

Developmental Abnormalities. Reflecting its noninvasive character, MRI is particularly well suited for the evaluation of congenital cardiovascular malformations of the aorta including arch anomalies and aortic coarctation. Contrast-enhanced 3D MRA can complement conventional MRI protocols by providing an accurate overview of the vascular morphology contained within a large 3D volume. Arch anomalies, such as a double aortic arch, aberrant left subclavian artery, right-sided aortic arch, and aortic pseudocoarctation are easily diagnosed. In the case of aortic coarctation the 3D MRA images do not merely display the

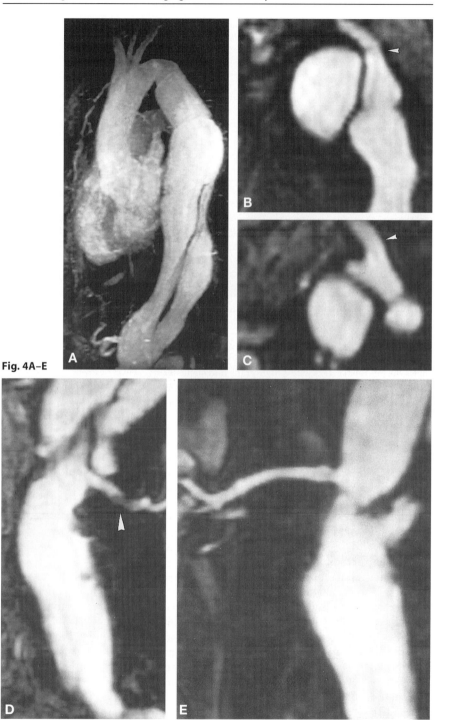

Fig. 4A–E

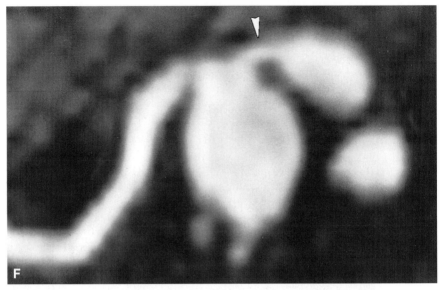

Fig. 4A–F. Follow-up MR examination following repair of a type B aortic dissection in a patient with Marfan Syndrome. Sagittal MIP (**A**) showing the short graft in the proximal descending aorta and aortic dissection with entry site in the distal descending aorta and a dissection membrane extending into the abdominal aorta. Axial reformatted images showing the celiac trunc (**B**) and SMA (**C**, *arrowheads*) arising from the false channel. Coronal reformatted image (**D**) shows the left renal artery with a high-grade mid stenosis (*arrowhead*). Coronal (**E**) and transverse (**F**) reformatted image shows the right renal artery arising from the true channel. A reentry tear (*arrowhead*) is also apparent at this level

exact location of the aortic stenosis but also provide information regarding the degree of luminal narrowing without the influence of spin-dephasing artifacts (Fig. 7). Collateral vessels bridging the stenosis, an important indicator of the hemodynamic significance of a lesion, are also well depicted on contrast-enhanced MR angiographic images (Fig. 7). Contrast-enhanced MRA is also useful for postoperative evaluation of patients following corrective surgical procedures (Fig. 8).

2.1.2.3 Extracranial Carotid Arteries
Due to the relatively high incidence of severe complications associated with selective catheter angiography of the carotid arterial system much interest has been generated in finding a noninvasive alternative for the preoperative evaluation of carotid bulb disease. Both duplex ultrasound and noncontrast MRA have been implicated as possible alternatives, but neither has provided the necessary accuracy in grading of stenoses. 3D contrast-enhanced MRA (Fig. 9) appears to be a promising method for the evaluation of extracranial carotid stenotic disease since it overcomes the limitations inherent to conventional MRA such as spin saturation and intravoxel phase dispersion thereby providing better depiction of the arterial lumen (Levy and Prince 1996).

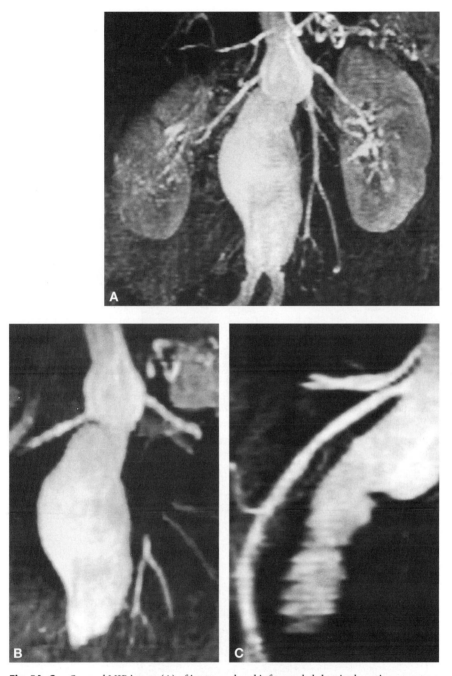

Fig. 5A–C. Coronal MIP image (**A**) of juxtarenal and infrarenal abdominal aortic aneurysms in a 56-year-old patient. Associated disease of the renal arteries the celiac trunk and superior mesenteric artery can be ruled out on coronal (**B**) and sagittal (**C**) reformatted images

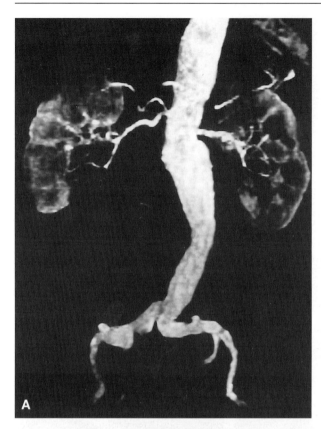

Fig. 6A, B. A 62-year-old patient with an infrarenal abdominal aortic aneurysm. Coronal MIP image (**A**) illustrates the aneurysmal lumen. Postcontrast transverse T1-weighted fat-suppressed SE image (**B**) demonstrates mural thrombosis and the true diameter of the aneurysm

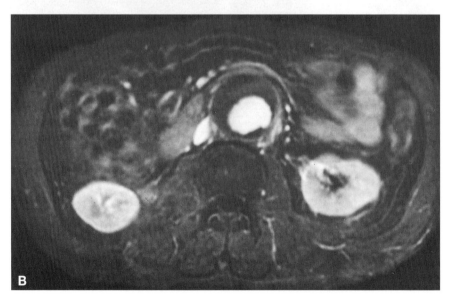

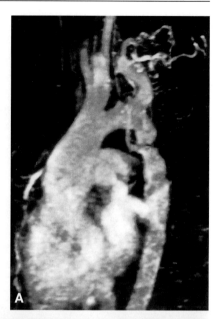

Fig. 7A, B.   A 24-year-old patient with aortic coarctation. Sagittal MIP image (**A**) depicting coarctation of the aorta with collateral vessels arising from the dilated left subclavian artery proximal to the stenosis. The extent of stenosis (**B**) is well visualized on reconstructed axial images of the 3D breath-hold contrast-enhanced MRA acquisition, depciting the descending aorta proximal to, within and distal to the coarctation.

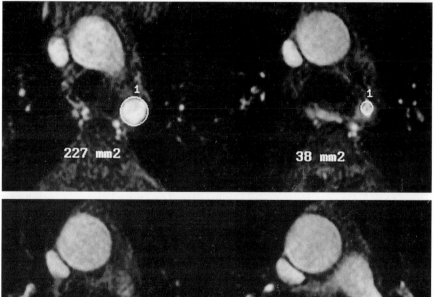

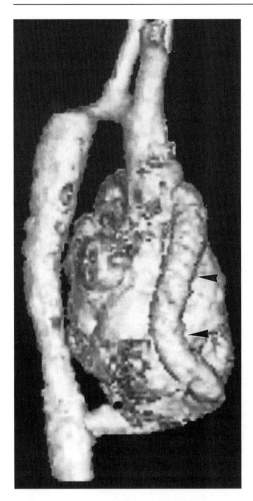

Fig. 8. Surface-shaded-display image of contrast-enhanced 3D MRA in a postoperative patient with aortic coarctation showing a bypass graft (*arrowhead*) connecting the ascending and descending aorta

The 3D MRA data can be acquired in the coronal or sagittal plane depending on the given arterial morphology of interest, thereby maximizing spatial resolution while minimizing imaging time (Fig. 10). The arterial-venous recirculation time in the carotid arteries is very short. As a result jugular venous enhancement is almost unavoidable and may obscure visualization of the adjacent carotid artery. Isolation of the arterial phase in the carotid arteries can however be assured by performing time-resolved 3D MRA (Korosoc et al., 1996).

The 3D nature of contrast-enhanced MRA allows image reformation in any plane, thus eliminating the possibility of projection-related misinterpretation of stenoses. This represents an advantage over conventional catheter angiography.

2.1.2.4 Renal Arteries

Renovascular disease may cause hypertension and/or ischemic nephropathy. Surgical or endovascular revascularization procedures are safe and reliable treat-

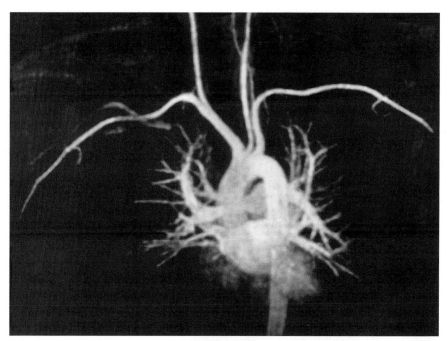

Fig. 9. MIP of 3D contrast-enhanced MRA in a healthy volunteer displaying the extracranial carotid and subclavian arteries to good advantage

ment options for both. Effective treatment, however, is predicated upon proper identification of patients with disease. Since clinical criteria for selecting patients are unreliable, radiographic screening techniques are highly desirable. Many such techniques have been developed including duplex sonography, intravenous digital subtraction angiography, and captopril radionuclide renography. Various limitations inherent to each one of these methods have prevented any one technique from establishing itself as the screening method of choice. Promising results have been demonstrated with helical CT angiography, but the need for large volumes of iodinated contrast has remained a barrier to its clinical acceptance, especially in patients with impaired renal function. Both TOF and PC MRA techniques have also been widely investigated as a possible tool for renal artery screening (Debatin et al. 1991; Servois et al. 1994). However, long imaging times, limited accuracy in grading of stenoses and the inability to reliably detect accessory renal arteries have prevented their widespread use.

Breath-hold contrast-enhanced 3D MRA is a promising new method for renal artery screening because it is fast, robust, non-operator-dependent, minimally invasive, and can be performed on patients with renal insufficiency. Since arterial contrast is not based on flow enhancement, overestimation of stenosis, a problem which has confounded traditional MR techniques, is no longer an issue. The accuracy of non-breath-hold contrast-enhanced MRA with respect to the

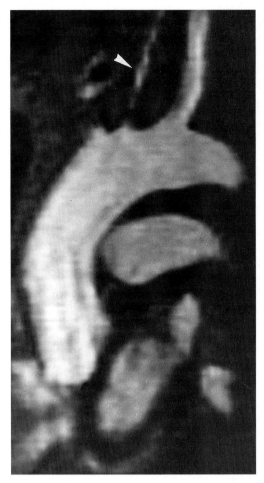

Fig. 10. A 58-year-old patient with extracranial carotid stenostic disease. Oblique reformatted image showing high grade stenosis of left common carotid artery with string sign (*arrowhead*) originating proximal to the left subclavian artery

grading of renal artery stenosis is limited by motion-induced blurring and the influence of enhanced overlapping veins. Prince (1994) reported a sensitivity and specificity of 85% and 93% for detection of renal artery stenosis while Kaufmann et al. (1994) reported a sensitivity and specificity of 89% and 98% for detection of stenoses of greater than 50%, albeit in a small sample. It has been shown that breath-hold data acquisition can significantly improve the visualization of renal arteries (Prince et al. 1995a,b). Indeed, Snidow et al. (1996) reported a sensitivity and specificity of 100% and 89% for detection of obstructive lesions of the renal arteries. In that study four of six false-positive diagnoses were caused by operator error or respiration, resulting in an unexpectedly low specificity. Our own experience (Hany et al. 1997a,e) with breath-hold contrast-enhanced MRA of the renal arteries in 49 patients yielded a sensitivity and specificity of 90% and 98% for diagnosis of lesions of greater than 50% and a detection rate of 100% for accessory renal arteries (Figs. 11, 12).

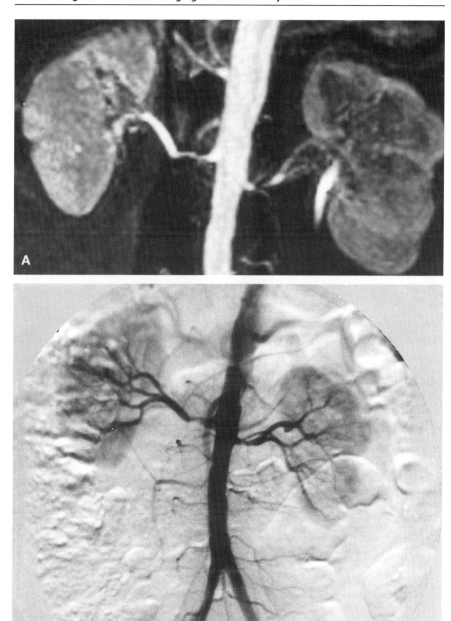

Fig. 11A, B. Atherosclerotic bilateral proximal renal artery stenosis in a 62-year-old patient with progressive renal insufficiency. The findings are displayed to similar advantage on the 3D contrast-enhanced MRA-MiP image (**A**) and the digital subtraction angiogram (**B**)

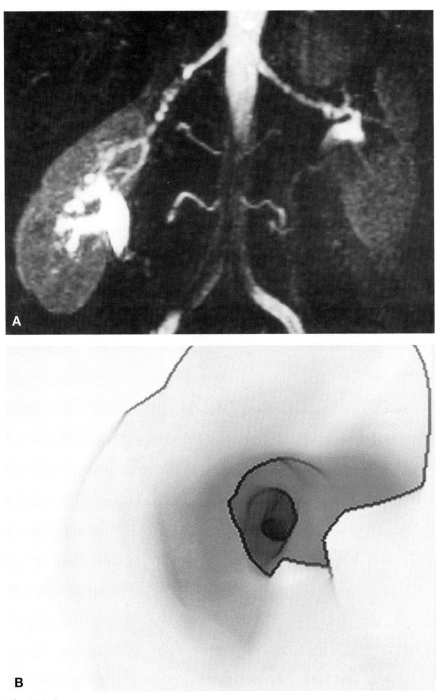

Fig. 12A, B

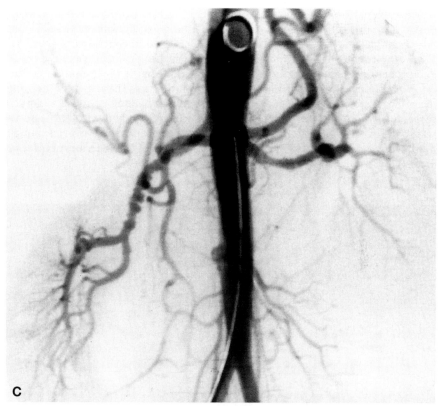

C

Fig. 12A–C. Bilateral fibromuscular dysplasia of the renal arteries in a 36-year-old hypertensive woman. Subvolume MIP image (**A**) depicts characteristic "string of beads." The virtual angioscopic view (**B**) from within the right renal artery demostrates the weblike stenoses. Findings are confirmed by the digital subtraction angiogram (**C**)

2.1.2.5 Celiac and Superior Mesenteric Arteries

Mesenteric ischemia remains a frequently perplexing diagnostic dilemma. Chronic mesenteric ischemia is caused by deficiency of blood supply to the intestine due to stenosis or occlusion of the splanchnic arteries. Despite the high incidence of celiac and mesenteric artery stenosis in patients with advanced atherosclerotic disease the syndrome of mesenteric ischemia is rare. This observation reflects the presence of a rich collateral network in the form of vascular arcades which readily compensate for stenosis or occlusion of a single splanchnic artery. Patients generally do not develop symptomatic mesenteric ischemia unless blood flow in at least two of the three visceral arteries is severely compromised. Duplex sonography has been suggested as a noninvasive screening test for patients with suspected mesenteric ischemia. Reliability and accuracy of duplex sonography is limited however by its inherent operator dependence. In addition, excess bowel gas and adipositas render a significant number of examinations nondiagnostic.

MRA and MR-based flow measurements have also been evaluated as diagnostic tests for ischemic bowel disease (Li et al. 1995; Burkart et al. 1995), but larger clinical studies are still outstanding. Breath-hold contrast-enhanced 3D MRA can provide rapid minimally invasive morphological assessment of celiac and superior mesenteric arteries (SMA; Fig. 13). Recently Meaney et al. (1997a) reported promising preliminary results in patients with suspected chronic mesenteric ischemia with sensitivity and specificity values of 100% and 95%, respectively. The authors concluded that 3D contrast-enhanced MRA is accurate in the evaluation of the origins of the mesenteric and celiac arteries though too low in image resolution for reliable assessment of the inferior mesenteric artery (Fig. 14).

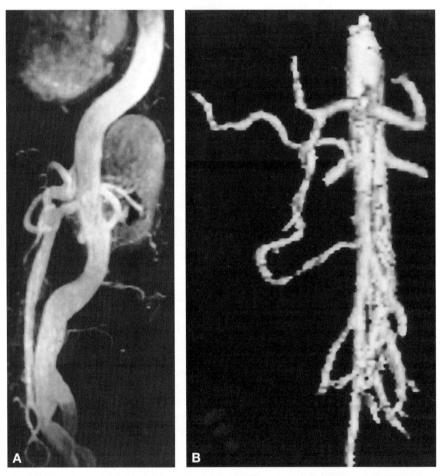

Fig. 13A, B. A 44-year-old patient with Marfan' syndrome. Sagittal MIP image (**A**) illustrates elongation of the aorta and a widely patent SMA. Coronal surface rendered display of the 3D data set (**B**) displaxs the branches of the celiac trunk and the SMA.

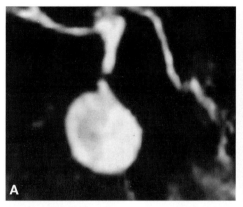
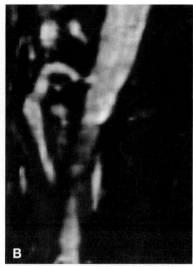
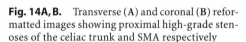

Fig. 14A, B.   Transverse (A) and coronal (B) reformatted images showing proximal high-grade stenoses of the celiac trunk and SMA respectively

2.1.2.6 Peripheral Arteries

Aortoiliac (Inflow Tract) Occlusive Disease.   Occlusive disease of the aortoiliac inflow tract usually affects the distal infrarenal aorta and the iliac arteries in smokers. Conventional angiographic evaluation of these patients generally involves both biplane catheter aortography and lower extremity arteriography. However, occlusion of the infrarenal aorta and/or iliac arteries due to atherosclerotic stenosis (Leriche syndrome), thromboembolism, occlusion of an aneurysm or iatrogenic causes is recognized as a distinct clinical entity and does not necessarily mandate imaging of the lower extremity runoff vessels if bilateral reconstitution can be demonstrated at or above the level of the external iliac arteries. In such patients 3D contrast-enhanced 3D MRA offers an attractive noninvasive alternative to transbrachial arteriography (Fig. 15). 3D MRA has a major impact in the presurgical evaluation of such patients because of the significant limitations of other noninvasive imaging techniques such as conventional 2D TOF MRA and duplex ultrsound. Indeed, several studies have demostrated the efficacy of 3D contrast-enhanced 3D MRA for the evaluation of obstructive lesions of the aorta and iliac arteries (Fig. 16), with sensitivities and specificities ranging from 90% to 100% (Snidow et al. 1996; Hany et al. 1997).

Femoropopliteal (Outflow Tract) Occlusive Disease.   Long imaging times, signal void associated with pulsatile flow in femoropopliteal arteries, and the inability to account for retrograde flow in collateral vessels characterize conventional 2D TOF methods for the evaluation of peripheral vascular disease. As a result stenoses tend to be overestimated, and the length of occlusions is difficult to assess. Moreover, conventional 2D TOF MRA lacks accuracy in the evaluation

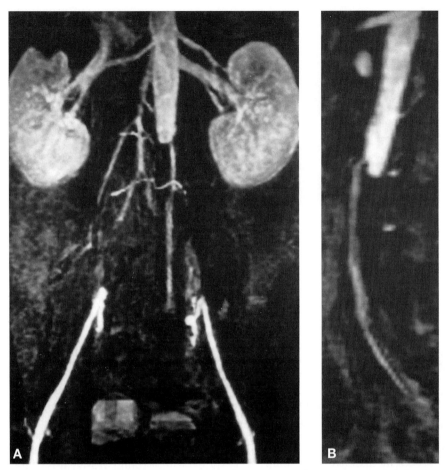

Fig. 15A, B. Leriche syndrome. A MIP image of 3D contrast-enhanced 3D MRA (**A**) showing aortic occlusion distal to the inferior mesenteric artery with bilateral reconstitution of blood flow in the distal common iliac arteries. Patent renal arteries and wedged-shaped perfusion defect in the upper pole of the right kidney is seen. (**B**) Sagittal reformatted image shows collateralization via the inferior mesenteric artery

of the pelvic arteries. The use of contrast-enhanced 3D MRA can potentially overcome many of these limitations (Fig. 17). However, new challenges arise, most notably the problem of covering the entire lower extremities. In its present form, 3D contrast-enhanced MRA does not offer comprehensive imaging of the arterial tree from the aortic bifurcation to the lower extremity runoff vessels. However, new contrast media (Fig. 18) and faster time-resolved data acquisition strategies (Korosec et al. 1996) may permit sequential angiographic evaluation at multiple stations with separate injections. Alternatively, the contrast bolus can be followed down into the legs, similarly as in conventional contrast arteriography. In the latter method asymmetric contrast travel time in the legs and delayed

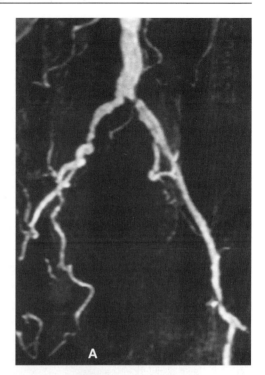

Fig. 16A, B.   MIP image of 3D contrast-enhanced 3D MRA (**A**) of a 56-year-old patient with peripheral vascular disease showing stenoses of the common iliac arteries and occlusion of the right common femoral artery. Conventional digital subtraction angiography (**B**) confirms MRA findings

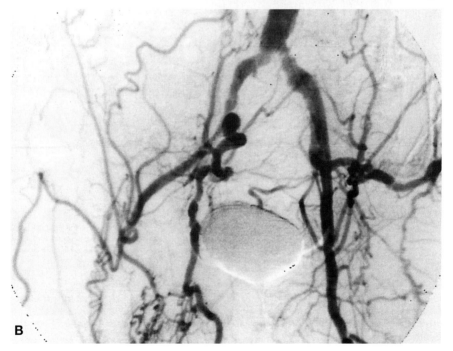

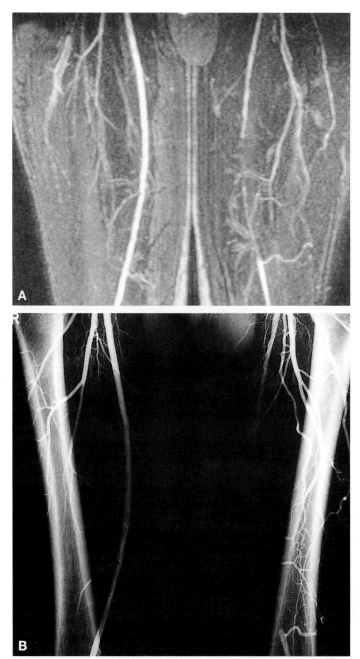

Fig. 17A, B.   MIP image of 3D contrast-enhanced 3D MRA (**A**) shows occlusion of the left superficial femoral artery. The length of the occlusion is easily assessed due to retrograde enhancement via collaterals from the deep femoral artery. Conventional angiography (**B**) confirms the findings

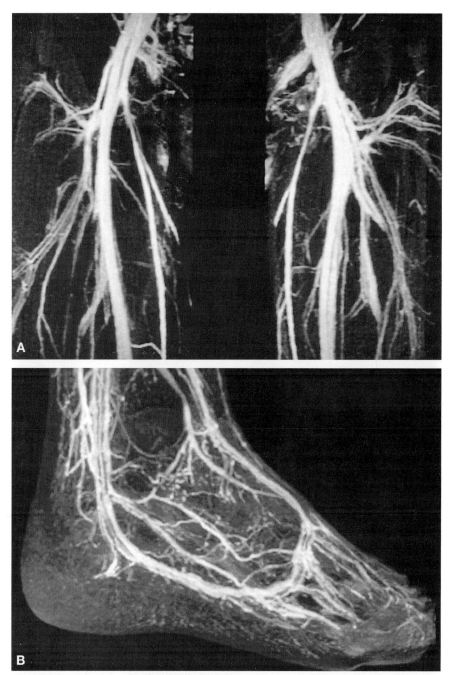

Fig. 18A, B. Contrast-enhanced MRA of the femoral arteries (**A**) and the arteries of the foot (**B**) in a healthy volunteer using a new intravascular contrast agent. (Nycomed Imaging, Oslo, Norway) Note intense enhancement of veins

enhancement distal to occlusions may present further challenges. Also here, the use of time resolved acquisition techniques (Korosec et al. 1996) which use a precontrast image as a subtractable mask will be essential for consistent results and to reduce contrast dose.

2.1.2.7 Portal Venous System

Contrast-enhanced 3D MRA allows exquisite morphological depiction of the portal venous system and the hepatic veins (Fig. 19). This is useful in the evaluation of patients with portal hypertension or portal venous thrombosis and in the pre- and posttherapeutic work-up of candidates for percutaneous or surgical portal-systemic shunt procedures or liver transplantation.

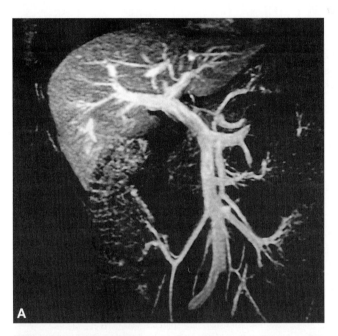

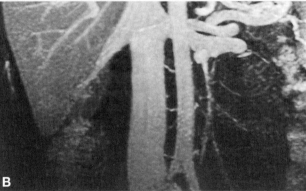

Fig. 19A, B. Breath-hold contrast-enhanced MRA projection images acquired 60 s following contrast administration depict the portal (**A**) and hepatic veins (**B**)

Imaging of the portal venous system with contrast-enhanced MRA can be performed either as a byproduct of abdominal aortic imaging simply by acquiring a second data set following the arterial phase or alternatively by measuring the contrast travel time to the portal vein and timing a single focused acquisition accordingly. With either method high-resolution images of the portal venous system are obtained. Despite increased dilution of the contrast agent in the venous system, the contrast-to-noise ratio of breath-hold contrast-enhanced portography is good and the technique offers better depiction of venous morphology than conventional noncontrast MRA. The direction of portal venous blood flow can be determined with PC MRA.

2.2   Echo-Planar MRA

Unlike contrast-enhanced 3D MRA, echo-planar MRA does not require the application of paramagnetic contrast agents. Similarly as in conventional MRA techniques, it relies on the display of flow phenomena. The technique continues to face considerable technical challenges and has thus remained largely experimental. As with other ultrafast techniques, the motivation behind the development of echo-planar MRA techniques is the reduction of motion artifacts by permitting breath-held data acquisition and improved temporal resolution to better characterize physiological motion patterns.

2.2.1   Technique Considerations

Options available for echo-planar MRA are similar to those of conventional MRA with respect to choice of pulse sequence. However, decisions must be tailored to meet the characteristics of the altered EPI environment. The first strategy decision pertains to which of the two basic vascular MRA approaches, TOF and PC, should be pursued. One of the more important factors favoring TOF over PC in conventional MRA is the length of the imaging time. Depending on whether flow is encoded in one or all three planes, PC data acquisition exceeds TOF imaging times by a factor of 2 or 4, respectively. With ultrafast EPI data collection techniques absolute differences in imaging times become considerably less relevant. Hence the advantages of PC imaging, including better stationary tissue supression, reduced intravoxel dephasing, reduced sensitivity to spin saturation and adjustable flow sensitivity (Applegate et al. 1992; Chao et al. 1989; Edelman 1993; Debatin et al. 1991; Spritzer et al. 1990; Huston and Ehman 1993) appear to outweigh those of TOF. Furthermore, the directional information inherent to PC imaging permits easy differentiation of venous from arterial signal, obviating the need for spatial saturation pulses.

Multiplanar cross-sectional acquisitions may be based on either 2D or 3D Fourier transforms. Although 2D approaches generally require less imaging time and are less sensitive to spin saturation phenomena, there are several advantages favoring a 3D approach. 3D MRA allows the acquisition of very thin sections with minimal interslice cross-talk (Wagle et al. 1989). The smaller voxel size reduces partial voluming errors and decreases intravoxel dephasing. These characteristics are of particular value in the assessment of the carotid bifurcation (Masaryk et al. 1991). 3D imaging is also characterized by higher SNR' values than 2D acquisitions. This makes the implementation of the 3D Fourier transform into SNR-limited echo-planar acquisition strategies a natural next step.

Another important reason favoring the use of 3D k-space acquisitions for echo-planar MRA reflects the pulsatility of the arterial system. The acquisition time for a 2D EPI image is considerably shorter than the length of an RR interval. To ensure that data collection coincides with maximal systolic flow image acquisition either needs to be gated to systole or, as suggested by Goldberg et al. (1993), multiple images need to be acquired in rapid succession in the same location. Both solutions result in a significant lengthening of imaging times, thus diminishing the speed advantage of EPI acquisitions. 3D EPI data sets, on the other hand, are collected over a period exceeding the length of several cardiac cycles; hence they represent flow averaged over that same period. This approach allows to take full advantage of EPI's ultrafast acquisition speed. For echo-planar MRA of the pulsatile arterial system a 3D scan thus appears to be the strategy of choice.

The understanding and correct interpretation of artifacts is a fundamental prerequisite to the clinical use of MRA. In general, the flow artifacts encountered in conventional MRA, including overestimation of the extent of stenoses, also apply to echo-planar MRA. With EPI, however, additional flow effects must be considered.

Motion in the section-select direction causes phase changes comparable to those of standard 2D Fourier transform acquisitions and does not produce additional artifacts. Hence, accurate through-plane flow measurements can be performed with EPI velocity mapping (McKinnon et al. 1994; Firmin et al. 1989). In-plane flow may result in spatial displacement due to the asynchronism of phase and the frequency-encoding gradients. This effect has been shown to be greater with EPI than with conventional sequences. Due to quadratic phase modulation (Wedeen et al. 1989) EPI images are also subject to blurring of vascular structures along the phase-encoding direction. As with the section select gradient, the phase-encoding gradient in blipped EPI acquisitions can be flow compensated, albeit only at one, generally the central k-space line (Butts and Riederer 1992). Flow compensation of all echoes is possible but increases imaging times by a factor of 2–3 (Duerk and Simonetti 1991). Due to even echo rephasing the flow in the frequency-encoding direction produces an additional phase shift on the odd gradient echoes. This causes ghosting, the severity of which depends on flow velocity (Butts and Riederer 1992). Multishot acquisitions cause multiple ghosts. These, however, are individually less intense than the ghosting artifacts seen in single-shot EPI.

EPI acquisitions are highly sensitive to susceptibility and chemical shift artifacts. Since the pixel bandwidth along the phase-encoding direction is much smaller than that along the frequency-encoding direction, these artifacts are propagated primarily in the phase-encoding direction. Owing to the relatively large fat shift with EPI, it is necessary to use fat suppression pulses or preferably spectral spatial excitation pulses (Meyer et al. 1990). As with the spatial distortions, chemical shift artifacts can be reduced by increasing the number of shots of the EPI acquisition.

2.2.2   Applications of echo-planar MRA

Unresolved technical challenges have hindered the implementation of echo-planar MRA in clinical practice (Debatin et al. 1995b). Potential benefits resulting from a significant reduction in data acquisition times combined with the display of vascular morphology without the use of expensive paramagnetic contrast agents, have, however, motivated the assessment of echo-planar MRA in a number of vascular territories, outlined below.

2.2.2.1 Carotid Arteries

In an attempt to reduce imaging times, an 8-shot echo-planar 3D PC sequence (Wildermuth et al. 1995) capable of collecting 64 sections with a thickness of 2.5 mm and an inplane resolution of 1×1 mm (26×13 cm FOV, 256×128 matrix) in merely 32 s, was implemented on a 1.5-T MRI system (Fig. 20). Comparable conventional strategies required 459 s to acquire the same amount of data. A direct comparison of echo-planar and conventional MRA image quality revealed similar performance of the two techniques in the proximal portion of the carotid arteries (common carotid artery, carotid bifurcation and the proximal internal and external carotid arteries; Fig. 21). Similarly, the proximal vertebral arterial segments were seen to equal advantage with both techniques. Due to increased spin dephasing, induced by a slightly longer echo time, the more distal arterial segments were less well seen with echo-planar compared to the conventional imaging technique.

Beyond increasing the number of signals averaged, the implementation of spatially variable flip angles, or TONE pulses (Purdy et al. 1992) or the acquisition of multiple thin slice 3D acquisitions (MOTSA; Blatter et al. 1991, 1992) might further improve the quality of EPI images. The administration of extracellular contrast agents would have a similar effect. EPI appears particularly well suited to take advantage of these extracellular agents as their half life in the vascular lumen is rather short. Contrast-enhanced MRA could hence be performed with conventional, already approved agents.

Even without these adjuncts limited patient experience suggests that this echo-planar MRA technique might indeed become useful as a screening tool for disease of at least the carotid bifurcation. The signal void caused by a high-grade stenosis in the proximal internal carotid artery reflects turbulent flow conditions and is similar in size to that seen in the conventionally acquired images. Good correlation with the invasive selective digital subtraction angiography is apparent. The very short data acquisition times allow the evaluation of this region as a quick adjunct to any MR evaluation of the head and neck. Further improvements in image quality coupled with thorough prospective studies examining the utility of this technique are warrented though, prior to any use of EPI MRA of the carotid and vertebral systems in a clinical setting.

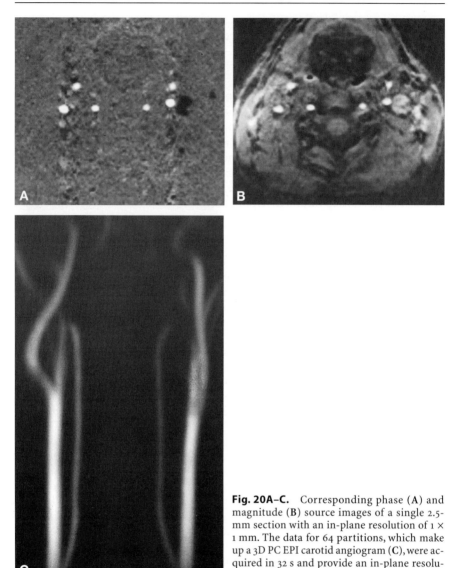

Fig. 20A–C. Corresponding phase (A) and magnitude (B) source images of a single 2.5-mm section with an in-plane resolution of 1 × 1 mm. The data for 64 partitions, which make up a 3D PC EPI carotid angiogram (C), were acquired in 32 s and provide an in-plane resolution of 1 × 1 mm.

2.2.2.2 Renal Arteries

A promising approach to renal arterial imaging with echo-planar MRA has been suggested by Wielopolski and Edelman (1994). They implemented a multishot EPI readout into the signal targeting with alternating radiofrequency (STAR) technique. The STAR technique is essentially a TOF subtraction method. The technique is based on a complex subtraction of two TOF data sets that differs solely by the signal from blood that has been selectively excited in one of the data sets.

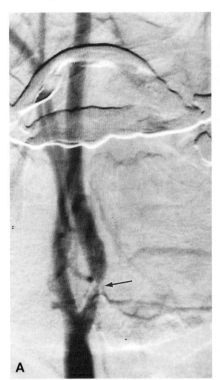
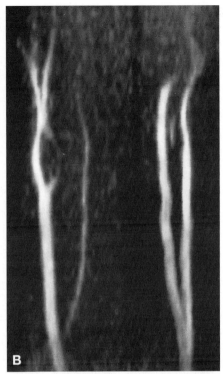

Fig. 21A, B. Selective digital subtraction angiogram (**A**) of the right carotid artery reveals a high-grade stenosis involving the proximal internal carotid artery (*arrow*) in a 63-year-old patient. The stenosis is identified on the echo-planar 3D PC MRA (**B**)

Using EPI STAR, magnetic resonance angiograms of the renal arteries have been obtained with excellent background suppression. Care must be taken to choose sections sufficiently thick to encompass all vessels of interest. The same group has implemented a 3D version of this technique, providing isotropic resolution and multiple views using the maximum intensity projection algorithms. Data with regard to the clinical performance of this technique are not yet available. Based on its performance in normal volunteers, it appears promising.

2.2.2.3 Trifurcation Arteries

Much attention has been centered on the performance of conventional MRA with regard to visualization of lower leg runoff vessels. MRA has actually been shown to be superior to conventional, invasive angiographic techniques with regard to identification of the distal runoff vessels in patients with severe proximal atherosclerotic disease (Owen et al. 1992). One of the problems limiting the broader clinical application of MRA for evaluation of peripheral atheroclerotic disease is the lengthy acquisition times. Additional problems arise with regard to suppression of venous flow. Travelling saturation bands must be applied. If they are

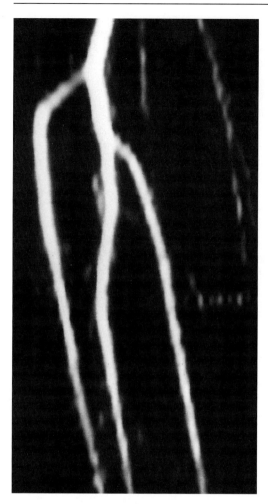

Fig. 22. MRA of the trifurcation arteries in a volunteer acquired with echo-planar 3D PC. The data set consists of 64 contiguous 3-mm sections with an in-plane resolution of 1.2 × 1.2 mm. The EPI data were acquired in only 19 s. Due to saturation effects the distal trifurcation vessels and branch vessels are only poorly seen

placed too close to the actual acquisition volume, the triphasic nature of the flow in the distal arteries might result in dark, bandlike artifacts. Placement of the saturation bands too far from the acquired section results in persistent venous signal degrading the quality of the resulting MR arteriogram.

The implementation of the above outlined multishot echo-planar 3D PC MRA technique overcomes both limitations: image acquisition time for 64 contiguous 3 mm sections is reduced to merely 19 s and the directional component inherent to PC imaging permits selective visualization of the arterial tree (Fig. 22). Initial comparisons between conventional 2D TOF and 3D EPI MRA of the trifurcation arteries in volunteers are encouraging (Holtz et al. 1996b). The EPI data were acquired following 2 min of arterial occlusion at the level of the thigh. With both techniques proximal portions of the trifurcation vessels were fully visualized. Distal vessels, however, were visualized to a lesser extent with the EPI technique,

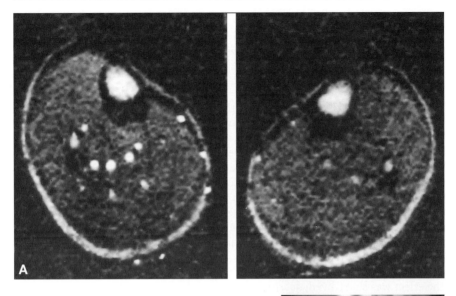

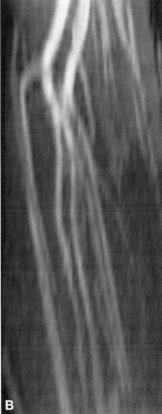

Fig. 23A, B. Forty-one axial contiguous 5-mm sections (**A**) through both calves make up the coronal projection MR EPI venogram (**B**). Data acquisition commenced immediately following termination of venous occlusion of the right thigh. Total imaging time for the entire acquisition was 10 s. Veins in the flow augmented right calf are well seen. Even small muscle veins are visualized reflecting in-volume dephasing due to the somewhat longer echo times. Similarly as in carotid echo-planar MRA, a variety of imaging options might vastly enhance the performance of this ultrafast data acquisition strategy for visualization of trifurcation arteries.

2.2.2.4 Calf Veins

Regardless of its origin, deep venous thrombosis of the lower extremities can embolize into the pulmonary arteries and cause significant morbidity and mortality (Barnes et al. 1989). The need for treatment mandates the identification of an accurate and preferably noninvasive diagnostic modality. Conventional MR venography has been shown to be as accurate as contrast venography and duplex ultrasound in the thigh, and superior to both techniques in the pelvis (Evans et al. 1993b). Evaluation of veins in the calf has remained challenging, reflecting the low velocity of blood flow within calf veins. Complete visualization of calf veins therefore appears contingent on an increase in flow velocity and thus intravascular signal intensity. A recent study (Holtz et al. 1996a) compared two mechanical flow augmenting measures – valsalva maneuver for 20 s and venous occlusion for 3 min. While both procedures significantly increased venous flow, the effect was short-lived, decreasing to normal values within 30 s.

The short-lived effects of mechanical flow augmentation can be exploited with ultrafast echo-planar data acquisition strategies (Holtz et al. 1996a). To provide adequate visualization of the small calf veins data acquisition was divided into four shots. Forty contiguous 5-mm 2D TOF sections were acquired in 10 s (Fig. 23). To maximize venous inflow effects the images were acquired from superior to inferior. Contamination of the venous signal by arterial flow was avoided by placing a superior spatial presaturation pulse, nulling signal in the arteries above the imaging volume. Since the technique is not based on retrograde contrast filling of the venous system, even small muscle veins draining into the deep veins can be visualized. (Fig. 23).

3 Vascular Function

MR techniques reach beyond the mere morphological assessment of the cardiovascular system by permitting direct quantitative characterization of flow dynamics (Pelc et al. 1991b). In analogy to MRA, both the influence of motion on signal amplitude and on signal phase can be exploited for flow measurements.

The amplitude technique exploits a TOF effect (Wehrli et al. 1986). It is based on the application of a thin saturation band across the vessel of interest and subsequent tracking the flow induced displacement of this band. This technique, referred to as bolus tracking, requires in-plane visualization of the vessel. While it has been shown accurately to measure flow velocities in large vessels such as the portal vein (Edelman et al. 1989a,b), the technique is handicapped by saturation phenomena, volume averaging, and insensitivity to slow flow.

The PC technique, on the other hand, provides velocity maps that directly determine the spatial mean velocity within each voxel across the lumen of a vessel.

By analyzing the vessel of interest in cross section it overcomes many of the limitations inherent to bolus tracking and Doppler ultrasound (Pelc et al. 1991a, b). This is particularly true with regard to flow volume quantitation, where Doppler ultrasound and MRI bolus tracking require determination of the vessel's diameter and assumptions with regard to the actual flow pattern within the interrogated vessel. Although the classification of flow dynamics seen in the vascular system has been subject to some controversy, there is general agreement that physiological velocity profiles usually constitute a mixture of different profiles (Caro et al. 1978). Modelling of in vivo flow is hence rather difficult and can potentially introduce considerable measurement error. Due to the pixel-based flow analysis inherent to MR phase mapping, the PC technique remains insulated from the ramifications of this discussion (Pelc et al. 1991a,b).

Following technical refinements in gradient and sequence design, the phase technique has thus emerged as the method of choice for flow quantitation with MRI (Haacke et al. 1991).

3.1 PC Mapping: Technical Considerations

PC MRI is based on the modulation of the phase of proton spins by varying the first moment of the magnetic field in any desired direction. A moment change causes spins moving in the encoded direction to acquire a phase shift which is directly proportional to velocity. Subtraction of two phase data sets acquired with different first moments along one direction produces a phase image reflecting information about motion in the encoded direction.

PC velocity data are temporal averages of instantaneous velocities. The degree of temporal averaging is determined by the length of the data acquisition window. For nongated sequences the latter is defined by the total imaging time. While this is sufficient for the quantitative characterization of constant flow found in much of the venous system, pulsatile arterial flow requires measurements at multiple points along the cardiac cycle.

Cine-PC imaging combines phase modulation with gradient echo cine-imaging. Pulse repetition is independent of the ECG signal, which is monitored and used to increment the spatial phase encoding at the beginning of each cardiac cycle retrospectively. For a single section and a single flow encoding direction two sequences with alternating first moments are interleaved during each cardiac cycle, yielding a two-dimensional, temporally resolved velocity map in a vascular cross section. Factors adversely affecting the accuracy of conventional cine-PC flow measurements include spatial and temporal averaging. These can be overcome with the implementation of ultrafast data collection stategies.

3.1.1 Spatial Averaging

Collection of cine-PC data is time consuming. Only a single k-line is acquired per RR interval for each of the cinematic frames spaced throughout the cardiac cycle. Thus even with limited spatial resolution minutes rather than seconds are required to collect a complete cine-PC data set.

Lengthy acquisition times prohibit data collection in apnea. In those thoracic and abdominal vessels with flow directions perpendicular to the respiration induced craniocaudad excursions, spatial averaging causes blurring of the target vessel resulting in overestimation of the apparent vessel size (Debatin et al. 1994). The extent of resultant overestimation of flow rate depends on the degree of motion relative to the vessel size (Debatin et al. 1994; Schoenenberger and Debatin 1996). In an in vitro simulation of respiratory effects on renal artery cine-PC flow measurements 5-mm excursions in the measurement plane at a rate of 12 min^{-1} caused a mean overestimation of true flow by 41.1% (Fig. 24; Debatin et al. 1994; Schoenenberger and Debatin 1996). Affected vessels include the coronary arteries, pulmonary arteries, portal vein, and renal arteries. For quantitative analysis of these, breath-held data acquisition strategies are clearly desirable.

To permit breath-held data acquisitions the PC technique has been implemented in segmented k-space acquisitions (Atkinson and Edelman 1991; Debatin et al. 1994; Fredrickson and Pelc 1994). These techniques use short repetition times around 5–10 ms. Several "bundled" phase encoding steps (views per segment) are acquired in rapid succession within each cardiac cycle. Since the bundled views in a single segment contribute to the reconstruction of the same phase image, the data acquisition time can be reduced by a factor correspond-

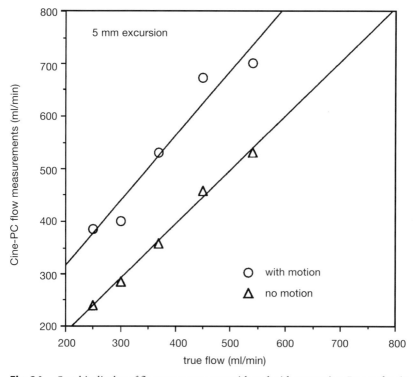

Fig. 24. Graphic display of flow measurements with and without motion. Due to the simulated respiratory motion, there is significant overestimation of flow in the phantom vessel

ing to the number of views per segment (generally 4–8), without sacrifice in spatial resolution. Segmented k-space acquisitions do permit data acquisition within a convenient breath-hold.

Compared to the retrospectively gated, slower Cine-PC technique, segmented PC acquisitions have several disadvantages however. Despite the use of very short TRs, the temporal resolution is sufficient only to collect between 4 and 12 quantitative data points throughout a cardiac cycle. The number of data points can be somewhat improved by employing "view-sharing", whereby new images are reconstructed based upon equal amounts of data from two neighboring images (Foo et al. 1993). The actual temporal resolution (ie., data acquisition time for an individual image), however, remains unaffected by this interpolation algorithm.

3.1.2 Temporal Averaging

The temporal resolution of conventional cine-PC sequences is defined by twice the length of the repetition time, amounting to as much as 60 ms (Pelc et al. 1991a, b). For segmented k-space sequences it is defined by twice the length of a "segment". The latter is determined by the TR, and the number of views per segment and can be as long as 150 ms. Thus the greater the number of views, the poorer is the temporal resolution.

The flow velocities displayed on the phase maps acquired with conventional or segmented k-space gradient echo sequences thus represent a rated average over the data-acquisition time for a single frame. Velocity averaging causes smoothing of peaks and troughs within flow cycles and precludes the assessment of dynamic flow responses to short-term cardiovascular challenges such as pharmacological stress or other factors directly affecting flow physiology. Hence flow volume measurements without sufficient temporal resolution may contain errors. These errors are unpredictable and may over- or underestimate true flow. Temporal resolution should therefore always be maximized providing

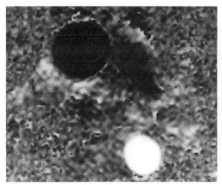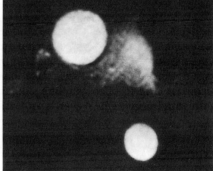

Fig. 25. Phase (left) and magnitude (right) images of a prospectively gated EPI-PC acquisition. Ascending and descending aorta are displayed at the level of the pulmonary bifuration. Over 9 heart beats sufficient data is collected to permit reconstruction of 24 phases within a cardiac cycle.

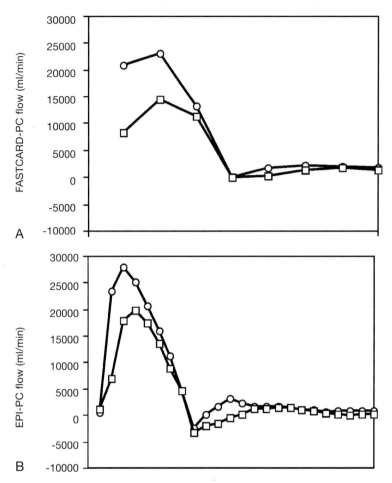

Fig. 26A, B. PC flow volume measurements of the ascending and descending aorta in the same volunteer are plotted over one cardiac cycle based on segmented k-space (FASTCARD) PC (**A**), and EPI PC (**B**) acquisitions. The limited temporal resolution of FASTCARD PC does not permit accurate definition of the triphasic aortic flow profiles. The EPI acquisition, on the other hand, provides sufficient temporal resolution to display the complex aortic flow patterns

at least 16–20 phases for flow quantification in highly pulsatile vessels such as the aorta or SMA.

To improve temporal resolution and still permit data collection in apnea, echo-planar data acquisition strategies (Debatin et al. 1995a) can be employed. Using a multishot echo-planar technique flow can be accurately quantitated both in vitro and in vivo (Debatin et al. 1995a,c; Figs. 25, 26). The technique provided as many as 24 phase images within a single cardiac cycle in a single breath-hold lasting merely 9 s. For quantitating flow in smaller vessels the technique remains handicapped however by poor spatial resolution and pulsatility artifacts.

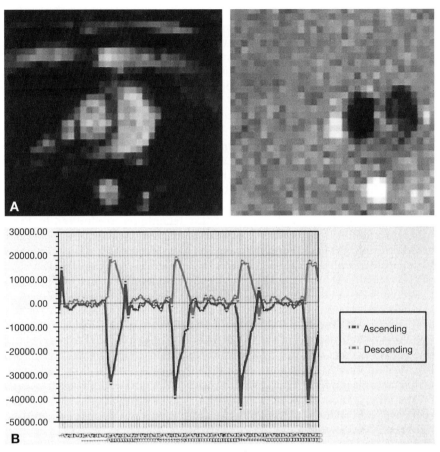

Fig. 27A, B. Single-shot EPI PC images acquired in real time are characterized by poor spatial resolution (A). The high temporal resolution does, however, permit characterization of flow profiles in the ascending and descending aorta relative to the respiratory cycle (B)

Truely real-time flow measurements can be achieved with single-shot PC EPI strategies (Eichenberger et al. 1995). Thus, flow profiles can be characterized within the aorta (Fig. 27) and the superior vena cava during the various forms of respiration.

3.2 Applications of Ultrafast PC Imaging

Quantitative PC flow mapping is a most powerful technique for assessing the functional component of flow throughout the vascular system. Conventional techniques, providing adequate spatial and temporal resolution, are time consuming but generally sufficient for most applications. Ultrafast data-acquisition strategies need to be employed if the PC measurements need to be performed in apnea. This is generally the case for all vessels subject to respiratory motion, particularly those with a flow direction perpendicular to the craniocaudad respiratory excursions. As examples for many possible applications of ultrafast PC sequences, the potential of renal and mesenteric arterial flow measurements is discussed in the following section. In both cases segmented k-space acquisitions are used.

3.2.1   Renal Arterial Flow Measurements

Compromise of renal arterial blood flow has long been recognized as a cause of hypertension (Hillman 1989) and end-stage renal disease (Rimmer and Gennari 1993). Most imaging methods hitherto employed rely on the morphological assessment of renal arteries. These techniques are limited by their inherent inability to predict the hemodynamic significance of a particular arterial lesion. PC flow mapping promises to overcome this deficit, by complementing morphological renal arterial MR imaging strategies (Debatin et al. 1994).

Prerequisite to any PC-based diagnosis of renovascular disease, however, is the ability to accurately quantitate renal arterial flow. In vitro and in vivo analyses have shown that accurate renal flow measurements are possible only if based upon breath-held data acquisitions (Debatin et al. 1994). Relative to renal blood flow measurements obtained by means of *para*-aminohippurate clearance, non-breath-held cine-PC imaging unpredictably overestimated flow, reflecting artifactual enlargement of the apparent vessel size. Accurate flow measurements, on the other hand, can be obtained with a time-resolved, segmented k-space sequence (Atkinson and Edelman 1991; Fredrickson and Pelc 1994), permitting the breath-held acquisition of six equally spaced PC frames in 37 s (Debatin et al. 1994).

It is important to acquire the PC data in a plane as perpendicular as possible to the vessel of interest. Ultrafast contrast-enhanced 3D MRA techniques (Leung et al. 1996) are well suited for a localizing roadmap displaying the exact 3D course of the renal arteries (Fig. 28). Due to the 3D nature of the data the correct scan plane, perpendicular to the renal artery and proximal to its first bifurcation, is easily identified. In addition, accessory renal arteries are readily seen. For accurate renal flow quantitation, it is important to measure flow in all vessels supplying a single kidney. Flow in supernumerary renal arteries must thus be measured as well (Fig. 29).

Renal arteries are characterized by a fairly homogeneous flow profile. Systolic peaks are low and diastolic flow is high, reflecting the retrograde flow component in the infrarenal aorta during diastole. In analogy to Doppler sonography, increases in systolic flow velocities associated with decreased diastolic flow have been associated with the presence of renal artery disease (Schoenberg et al. 1996). Although preliminary results appear promising, the significantly poorer temporal resolution of PC MRI compared to Doppler sonography casts a shadow of doubt over velocity-based analysis of renal flow profiles.

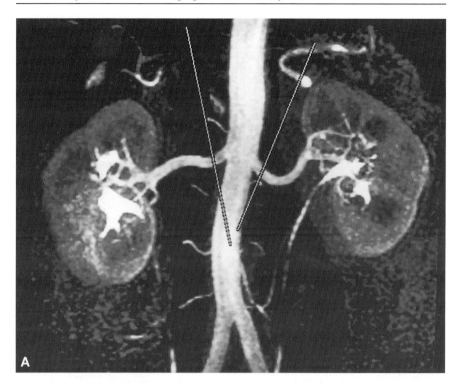

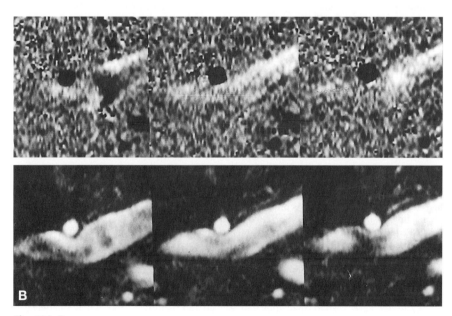

Fig. 28A, B

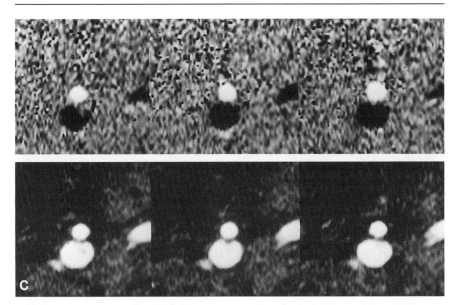

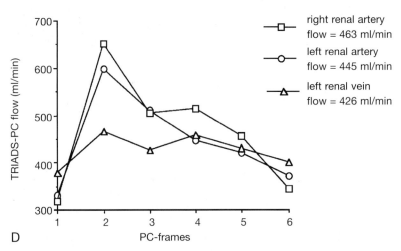

Fig. 28A–D. (**A**) MIP projection of a contrast-enhanced 3D MRA displaying normal renal arteries. The 3D data set consists of 44 contiguous 2-mm sections collected over a convenient breath-hold lasting 23 s. The 3D morphological images are well suited as a basis for planning the PC acquisition transsecting the renal artery in a plane perpendicular to its course and proximal to the take-off of the first branch vessel. Breath held segmented k-space PC acquisitions acquired perpendicular to the left (**B**) and right renal artery (**C**) show the magnitude images on top and the corresponding PC images on the bottom. Based on their respective flow directions the left renal artery (*arrow*) is displayed bright, while the left renal vein and right renal artery are shown as *black* on the PC images. Renal flow volumes of this subject are plotted over a cardiac cycle (**D**). There is good correlation between left and right renal arterial flow and between left arterial and left venous flow

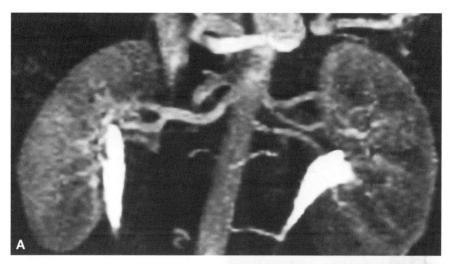

Fig. 29A–C. (A) MIP projection of a contrast-enhanced 3D MRA displaying three normal renal arteries on the left and a single vessel on the right. (B) For accurate renal flow quantitation, flow must be measured in all vessels supplying one kidney. The three arterial vessels are labeled. If the course of the accessory arteries is not parallal, a different PC acquisition needs to be planned for each. (C) The flow volume is plotted for all three left-sided renal arteries over a single cardiac cycle

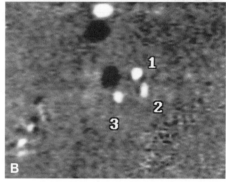

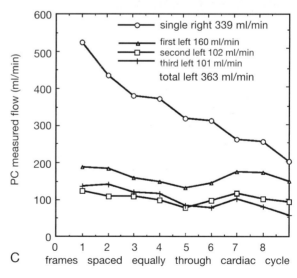

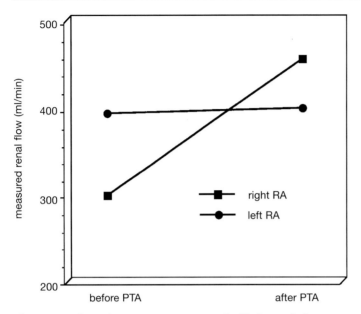

Fig. 30. PC flow volume measurements acquired before and after percutaneous transluminal angioplasty (*PTA*) reveals a vast PTA-induced increase in renal flow volume in the right renal artery (RA).

In addition to the ability of any other noninvasive technique including Doppler sonography, PC MRI can accurately quantitate renal arterial flow volume. Due to the inherent anatomic variance in renal position and size, the value of absolute flow volume numbers is limited. Two measurements over time, however, permit relative comparisons. Thus the therapeutic effect of various interventions such as percutaneous transluminal angioplasty (PTA) can be quantitated (Fig. 30). Furthermore, the effect of various vasoactive agents onto renal arterial flow volume can be measured with PC flow mapping. Initial work with amino acids and dobutamine has clearly demonstrated the ability of breathheld renal PC measurements to characterize even subtle pharmacological effects (Debatin et al. 1994).

Renal blood volume can also be related to renal tissue volume. In a recent study renal flow volumes were determined with PC MRI in 20 patients containing 40 kidneys. Arterial flow was normal in 28 kidneys and impaired due to the presence of a stenosis in 12 kidneys (G. Zimmermann 1997), personal communication). Analysis of the flow volume data reveals a significant difference between kidneys with normal arterial flow and those with impaired arterial supply (Fig. 31). These data suggest the existence of a critical cutoff value beyond which renal ischemia is indeed induced. Such a value may be able to aid in the differentiation between hemodynamically significant and nonsignificant renal arterial disease. Clearly further study is warranted to explore this exciting quantitative means for assessing renovascular disease.

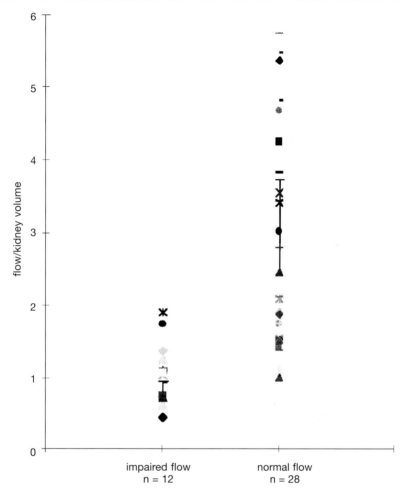

Fig. 31. Scatter diagram plotting renal flow volumes per renal mass (ml/cm^3). A significant difference ($p < 0.05$) is seen in renal flow between kidneys with impaired arterial flow, and those with normal arterial supply. There remains, however, some overlap (G. Zimmerman 1997, personal communication)

3.2.2   Mesenteric Ischemia

Due to the risks associated with arterial catheterization, the clinical diagnosis of mesenteric ischemia is generally one of exclusion. Delays in diagnosis are compounded by the propensity for symptoms of mesenteric ischemia to overlap with and mimic those of more common intestinal disorders such as peptic ulcer disease, chronic cholecystitis, and pancreatic carcinoma. Establishing the diagnosis of mesenteric ischemia is highly desirable, however, as surgical endarterectomy, reimplantation or transluminal angioplasty of the diseased vessels offer

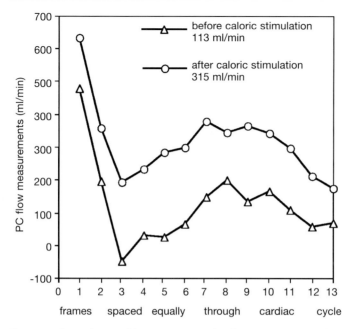

Fig. 32. Flow volumes of the SMA measured with PC MRI over a cardiac cycle in a healthy volunteer before and following stimulation with a standard (475 kcal) meal. Following caloric stimulation flow increased 80% relative to the fasting baseline

primary success rates varying between 80%–100% and 50%–75% for long-term clinical improvement.

Ultrafast breath-held PC MRI has been employed to assess flow volumes in the SMA and superior mesenteric vein (SMV; Li et al. 1994). To avoid respiratory motion, flow measurements of the SMA should be performed close to the vessel's origin. For maximal diagnostic efficacy measurements should be made both in the fasting state and following caloric stimulation. Postprandial flow in the SMA has been shown to increase over 100% in normal volunteers (Schoenenberger et al. 1996; Fig. 32). This postprandial hyperemia was significantly reduced (51%) in a patient with high-grade (> 50%) stenosis (Li et al. 1994). The percentage change in SMA blood flow 30 min after food intake provided the best distinction between healthy subjects, asymptomatic and symptomatic patients. In a limited number of patients with hemodynamically less significant stenoses (> 50%) the postprandial flow increase was indistinguishable from that seen in normal volunteers. The same investigators reported that increased postprandial blood flow within the SMV out of proportion to SMA blood flow is another marker for mesenteric ischemia. Discrepantly increased SMV flow reflects recruitment of collateral flow, induced by the presence of a significant SMA stenosis (Li et al. 1994).

References

Applegate GR, Talagala SL, Applegate LJ (1992) MR angiography of the head and neck: value of two-dimensional phase-contrast projection technique. AJR 159:369–374

Atkinson DJ, Edelman RR (1991) Cineangiography of the heart in a single breath hold with a segmented turboFLASH sequence. Radiology 178:357–360

Barnes RW, Nix ML, Barnes CL (1989) Perioperative asymptomatic venous thrombosis: role of duplex scanning versus venography. J Vasc Surg 9:251–260

Blatter DD, Parker DL, Robison RO (1991) Cerebral MR angiography with multiple overlapping thin slab acquisition. I. Quantitative analysis of vessel visibility. Radiology 179:805–811

Blatter DD, Parker DL, Ahn SS, Bahr AL, Robison RO, Schwartz RB, Jolesz FA, Boyer RS (1992) Cerebral MR angiography with multiple overlapping thin slab acquisition. II. Early clinical experience. Radiology 183:379–389

Burkart DJ, Johnson CD, Reading CC, Ehman RL (1995) MR measurements of mesenteric venous flow: prospective evaluation in healthy volunteers and patients with suspected chronic mesenteric ischemia. Radiology 194:801–806

Butts K, Riederer SJ (1992) Analysis of flow effects in echo-planar imaging. JMRI 2:285–293

Caro CG, Pedley TJ, Schroter RC, Seed WA (1978) The mechanics of the circulation. Oxford University Press, New York

Chao PW, Goldberg H, Dumoulin CL, Wehrli FW (1989) Comparison of time of flight versus phase contrast techniques: visualization of the intra and extracerebral carotid artery. In: Society of Magnetic Resonance in Medicine (ed) Book of abstracts. Society of Magnetic Resonance in Medicine, Amsterdam, p 165

Debatin JF, Spritzer CE, Grist TM, Beam C, Svetkey L, Newman GE, Sostman HD (1991) Imaging of the renal arteries: value of MR angiography. AJR 157:981–990

Debatin JF, Ting RH, Wegmüller H, Sommer FG, Fredrickson JO, Brosnan TJ, Bowman BS, Myers BD, Herfkens RJ, Pelc NJ (1994) Renal artery blood flow: quantification with phase contrast imaging with and without breath-holding. Radiology 190:371–378

Debatin JF, Davis CP, Felblinger J, McKinnon GC (1995a) Evaluation of ultrafast phase contrast imaging in the thoracic aorta. Magma 3:59–66

Debatin JF, Leung DA, Wildermuth S, Holtz D, McKinnon GC (1995b) Advances in vascular echoplanar imaging. Cardiovasc Intervent Radiol 18:277–287

Debatin JF, Wildermuth S, Leung DA, Botnar R, Felblinger J, McKinnon GC (1995c) Flow quantitation with echo-planar phase-contrast velocity mapping: in vitro and in vivo evaluation. JMRI 5:656–662

Duerk JL, Simonetti OP (1991) Theoretical aspects of motion sensitivity and compensation in echo-planar imaging. JMRI 1:643–650

Edelman RR (1993) MR angiography: present and future. AJR 161:1–11

Edelman RR, Mattle HP, Kleefield J, Silver MS (1989a) Quantification of blood flow with dynamic MR imaging and presaturation bolus tracking. Radiology 171:551–556

Edelman RR, Zhao B, Liu C, Wentz KU, Mattle HP, Finn JP, McArdle C (1989b) MR angiography and dynamic flow evaluation of the portal venous system. AJR 153:755–760

Eichenberger AC, Schwitter J, McKinnon GC, Debatin JF, von Schulthess GK (1995) Phase contrast echo planar MRI: real time quantification of flow and velocity patterns in the thoracic vessels induced by Valsalva's maneuver. J Magn Reson Imaging 5:648–655

Evans AJ, Iwai F, Grist TA et al (1993a) Magnetic resonance imaging of blood flow with a phase subtraction technique: 'in vitro' and 'in vivo' validation. Invest Radiol 28:109–115

Evans AJ, Sostman HD, Knelson MH, Coleman RE, Grist TM, MacFall JR (1993b) Detection of deep venous thrombosis: Prospective comparison of MR imaging with contrast venography. AJR; 161:131–139

Firmin DN, Klipstein RH, Hounsfield GL, Paley MP, Longmore DB (1989) Echo-planar high-resolution flow velocity mapping. Magn Reson Med 12:316–327

Foo TKF, McFall JR, Hayes CE, Sostman HD, Slayman BE (1992) Pulmonary vasculature: single breath-hold MR imaging with phased-array coils. Radiology 183: 473–477

Foo TK, Bernstein T, Aisen A, Hernandez RJ, Collick BD, Pavlik G (1993) High temporal resolution breath-held cine cardiac imaging using view sharing. In: Society of Magnetic Resonance in Medicine (ed) Book of abstracts. Society of Magnetic Resonance in Medicine, Amsterdam, p 1269

Fredrickson JO, Pelc NJ (1994) Time-resolved MR imaging by automatic data segmentation. JMRI 4:189–196

Galanski M, Prokop M, Chavan A, Schaefer CM, Jandeleit K, Nischelsky JE (1993) Renal artery stenosis: CT angiography. Radiology 189:185–192

Goldberg MA, Yucel EK, Saini S, Hahn PF, Kaufman JA, Cohen MS (1993) MR angiography of the portal and hepatic venous systems: preliminary experience with echoplanar imaging. AJR 160:35–40

Haacke EM, Smith AS, Lin W, Lewin JS, Finelli DA, Duerk JL (1991) Velocity quantification in magnetic resonance imaging. Magn Reson Imaging 3:34–49

Hany TF, Debatin JF, Leung DA, Pfammatter T (1997a) Evaluation of the aortoiliac and renal arteries with breath-hold contrast-enhanced 3D MR angiography: comparison with conventional angiography. Radiology 204:357–362

Hany TF, McKinnon GC, Leung DA, Pfammatter T, Debatin JF (1997b) Optimization of contrast timing for breathhold 3D MR angiography. JMRI 7:551–556

Hany TF, Schmidt M, Steiner P, Debatin JF (1997c) Optimization of Contrast Dosage for Gadolinium-Enhanced 3d MRA of the Pulmonary and Renal Arteries. Mag. Res. Imaging (in press)

Hany TF, Schmidt M, Davis CP, Göhde SC, Debatin JF (1997d) Diagnostic Impact of four Different Post-Processing Techniques in the Evaluation of Contrast-Enhanced 3D MR Angiography; AJR (in press)

Hany TF, Pfammatter T, Schmidt M, Leung DA, Debatin JF (1997e) Ultraschnelle, Kontrastverstärkte 3D MR-Angiographie der Aorta und Nierenarterien in Apnoe. RoFo; 166.5: 397-405

Holtz DJ, Debatin JF, McKinnon GC, Unterweger M, Wildermuth S, Fuchs WA (1996a) MR venography of the calf: vlaue of flow-enhanced time-of-flight echoplanar imaging. Am J Radiol 166:663–668

Holtz DJ, Unterweger M, McKinnon GC, Wildermuth S, Leung DA, von Schulthess GK, Debatin JF (1996b) Combining echo planar techniques with local flow-enhancing maneuvers: a new strategy for ultrafast MR imaging of calf arteries and veins. J Vasc Invest 2(3):118–124

Hillman BJ (1989) Imaging advances in the diagnosis of renovascular hypertension. AJR 153:5–14

Huston J III, Ehman RL (1993) Comparison of time-of-flight and phase-contrast MR neuroangiographic techniques. Radiographics 13:5–19

Kaufmann JA, Geller SC, Petersen MJ, Cambria RP, Prince MR, Waltman AC (1994) MR imaging (including MR angiography) of abdominal aortic aneurysms: comparison with conventional angiography. AJR 163:203–210

Korosec FR, Frayne R, Grist TM, Mistretta CA (1996) Time-resolved contrast-enhanced 3D MR angiography. Magn Reson Med 36:345–351

Leung DA, McKinnon GC, Davis CP, Pfammatter T, Krestin GP, Debatin JF (1996) Breathheld contrast-enhanced 3D MR angiography. Radiology 201:569–571

Leung DA, Debatin JF (1997) Three-Dimensional Contrast-Enhanced MRA of the thoracic Vasculature. Eur. Radiology; 7:981–989

Levy R, Prince MR (1996) Arterial-phase three-dimensional contrast-enhanced MR angiography of the carotid arteries. AJR 167:211–215

Li KCP, Whitney WS, McDonnell CH, Fredrickson JO, Pelc NJ, Dalman RL, Jeffrey RB Jr (1994) Chronic mesenteric ischemia: evaluation with phase-contrast cine MR imaging. Radiology 190:175–179

Li KCP, Hopkins KL, Dalman RL, Song CK (1995) Simultaneous measurement of flow in the superior mesenteric vein and artery with cine phase-contrast MR imaging: value in diagnosis of chronic mesenteric ischemia. Radiology 194:327–330

Mansfield P (1977) Multiplanar image formation using NMR spin-echoes. J Phys C Solid State Phys 10:L55–L58

Masaryk AM, Ross JS, Di Cello MC, Modic MT, Paranandi L, Masaryk TJ (1991) 3DFT MR angiography of the carotid bifurcation: potential and limitations as a screening examination. Radiology 179:797–804

McKinnon GC, Debatin JF, Wetter DR, von Schulthess GK (1994) Interleaved echo planar flow quantitation. Magn Reson Med 32:1–5

Meaney JFM, Prince MR, Nostrant TT, Stanley JC (1997a) Gadolinium-enhanced MR angiography of the visceral arteries in patients with suspected chronic mesenteric ischemia. JMRI 7:171–176

Meaney JFM, Weg JG, Chenervet TL, Stafford-Johnson D, Hamilton BH, Prince MR (1997b) Diagnosis of pulmonary embolism with magnetic resonance angiography. N Engl J Med 336:1422–1427

Meyer CH, Pauly JM, Macovski A, Nishimura DG (1990) Simultaneous spatial and spectral selective excitation. Magn Reson Med 15:287–304

Niendorf HP, Haustein J, Cornelius I, Alhassan A, Clauss W (1991) Safety of gadolinium-DTPA: extended clinical experience. Magn Reson Med 22:222–228

Owen RS, Carpenter JP, Baum RA, Perloff LJ, Cope C (1992) Magnetic resonance imaging of angiographically occult runoff vessels in peripheral arterial occlusive disease. N Engl J Med 326:1577–1581

Pelc NJ, Bernstein M, Shimakawa A, Glover G (1991a) Encoding Strategies for three-direction phase contrast MR imaging of flow. JMRI 1:405–413

Pelc NJ, Herfkens RJ, Shimakawa A, Enzmann DR (1991b) Phase contrast cine magnetic resonance imaging. Magn Reson Q 7:229–254

Prince MR (1994) Gadolinium-enhanced MR aortography. Radiology 191:155–164

Prince MR, Yucel EK, Kaufmann JA, Harrison DC, Geller SC (1993) Dynamic gadolinium-enhanced three dimensional abdominal MR arteriography. JMRI 3:877–881

Prince MR, Narasimhan DL, Stanley JC et al (1995a) Breath-hold gadolinium-enhanced MR angiography of the abdominal aorta and its major branches. Radiology 197:785–792

Prince MR, Narasimham DL, Stanley JC, Wakefield TW, Messina LM, Zelenock GB, Jacoby WT, Marx MV, Williams DM, Cho KJ (1995b) Gadolonium-enhanced magnetic resonance angiography of abdominal aortic aneurysms. J Vasc 21:656–69

Prince MR, Narasimhan DL, Jacoby WT et al (1996) Three-dimensional gadolinium-enhanced MR angiography of the thoracic aorta. Am J Roentgenol 166:1387–1397

Purdy DE, Cadena G, Laub G (1992) Variable-tip-angle slab selection for improved three-dimensional MR angiography. In: Society of Magnetic Resonance in Medicine (ed) Book of abstracts. Society of Magnetic Resonance in Medicine, Berlin, p 882

Rimmer JM, Gennari FJ (1993) Atherosclerotic renovascular disease and progressive renal failure. Ann Intern Med 118:712–719

Rubin GD, Walker PJ, Dake MD et al (1994) Three-dimensional spiral computed tomographic angiography: an alternative imaging modality for the abdominal aorta and its branches. J Vasc Surg 18:656–664

Schoenberg S, Knopp MV, Bock M, Kallinowski F, Just A, van Kaick G (1996) MR flow measurements for different of renal artery stenosis. In: International Society of Magnetic Resonance in Medicine (ed) Book of Abstracts. International Society of Magnetic Resonance in Medicine, New York, p 164

Schoenenberger A, Debatin JF (1996) Einfluss von Atmung und Pulsatilität auf die Genauigkeit von MR Phasenkontrast-Messungen: 'In Vitro' Evaluationen. RoFo 165(2):130–136

Schoenenberger AW, Hany TF, Ladd ME, McKinon GC, Debatin JF (1996) Angiography of the superior mesenteric artery: flow quantitation and clinical validation. Radiology 201(P):377

Servois V, Laissy JP, Feger C, Sibert A, Delahousse M, Baleynaud S, Mery JP, Menu Y (1994) Two-dimensional time-of-flight magnetic resonance angiography of renal arteries without maximum intensity projection: a prospective comparison with angiography in 21 patients screened for renovascular hypertension. Cardiovasc Intervent Radiol 17:138–142

Snidow JJ, Johnson MS, Harris VJ, Margosian PM, Aisen AM, Lalka SG, Cikrit DF, Trerotola SO (1996) Three-dimensional gadoloium-enhanced MR angiography for aortoiliac inflow assessment plus renal artery screening in a single breath hold. Radiology 198:725–732

Spritzer CE, Pelc NJ, Lee JN, Evans AJ, Sostman HD, Riederer SJ (1990) Rapid MR imaging of blood flow with a phase-sensitive, limited-flip-angle, gradient recalled pulse sequence: preliminary experience. Radiology 176:255–262

Steiner P, McKinnon GC, Romanowski B, Goehde SC, Hany TF, Debatin JF (1997) Contrast-enhanced, ultrafast 3D pulmonary MR angiography in a single breath-hold: initial assessment of imaging performance. JMRI 7:177–182

Wagle WA, Dumoulin CL, Souza SP, Cline HE (1989) 3DFT MR angiography of carotid and basilar arteries. AJNR 10:911–919

Wedeen VJ, Wedt RE, Jerosch-Herold M (1989) Motional phase artifacts in Fourier transform MRI. Magn Reson Med 11:114–120

Wehrli FW, Shimakawa A, Gullberg GT, MacFall JR (1986) Time-of-flight MR flow imaging: selective saturation recovery with gradient refocussing. Radiology 160:781–785

Wielopolski PA, Edelman RR (1994) Ultrafast, high resolution 3D STAR MR angiography using interleaved segmented echo planar readouts. In: Society of Magnetic Resonance (ed) Book of abstracts. Society of Magnetic Resonance, San Francisco, p 948

Wielopolski PA, Haacke EM, Adler LP (1992) Venous-suppressed pulmonary vasculature: preliminary experience. Radiology 183:465–472

Wildermuth S, Debatin JF, Huisman TAGM, Leung DA, McKinnon GC (1995) 3D phase contrast EPI MR-angiography of the carotid arteries. J Comput Assist Tomogr 19(6):871–878

5 Ultrafast Magnetic Resonance Imaging of the Abdomen

S. C. Göhde and J. F. Debatin

1 Introduction

Peristalsis, pulsatility, and respiratory motion have limited the use of magnetic resonance imaging (MRI) in the evaluation of abdominal pathology. The long imaging times of conventional spin-echo (SE) imaging precluded data acquisition in apnea. To overcome respiratory motion various compensation and triggering algorithms were developed and implemented. Flow compensation and the placement of spatial presaturation bands were recommended to reduce pulsatility artifacts. The use of glucagon has been suggested to reduce peristaltic bowel motion. In addition, multiple signals were averaged. The effect of these extensive efforts remained limited as they frequently resulted in blurring (Saini and Nelson 1995). As a result the diagnostic performance of MRI remained at par or slightly below that of computed tomography (CT). In the evaluation of colorectal cancer, pancreatic adenocarcinoma, and hepatocellular cancers (Zerhouni et al. 1996; Wernecke et al. 1991; Megibow et al. 1995) the superior soft tissue contrast of MRI was not sufficient to compensate for the persistent motion-induced artifacts degrading image quality.

The availability of fast and ultrafast data-acquisition strategies has effectively overcome many of these limitations by permitting the collection of entire MR data sets in apnea. The considerable ensuing improvements in image quality quickly translated into improved diagnostic performance of MRI compared to CT in the assessment of parenchymal abdominal organs (Semelka et al. 1992a,b, 1993a,b). This chapter focuses on the use of fast (turbo) SE and inversion recovery sequences and the widespread application of T1-weighted gradient-recalled echo (GRE) sequences before and following intravenous administration of paramagnetic contrast. Phase-shift GRE techniques for characterization of adrenal lesions are covered as well as the potential of ultrafast 3D data-acquisition strategies permitting the collection of an entire 3D data set within a single breath-hold for imaging of the stomach and colon. Finally, experimental work using echo-planar data-acquisition strategies is discussed.

2 Fast (Turbo) T2-Weighted Imaging

2.1 Technique Considerations

Contrast differences based upon T2 relaxation times have been shown to be most useful in the assessment of abdominal pathology. Long T2 relaxation times of water make T2-weighted sequences sensitive to the detection of cysts and tissue edema. Signal intensities on T2-weighted images have even been used for characterizing mass lesions as benign or malignant. The sensitivity to water can be enhanced by using an inversion pulse with a short inversion time to null the signal of fat. This is the basis of STIR sequences.

Both conventional T2-weighted SE and STIR imaging have, however, been handicapped by long data-acquisition times and associated motion artifacts. The implementation of RARE data-acquisition techniques (see Chap. 1) has contributed to a considerable shortening of imaging times and to a reduction in artifacts.

2.1.1   T2-Weighted Spin-Echo Sequence

All SE sequences consist of a combined 90° and 180° pulse. The initial 90° pulse flips the z-magnetization into the xy-plane. The resultant xy-magnetization subsequently decays with the transverse relaxation time constant T2. T2* effects, induced by external field inhomogeneities, are reversed by the 180° pulse. Long acquisition times make the sequence subject to motion artifacts. Their adverse effects on image quality can be limited by various compensation algorithms.

Respiratory artifacts can be reduced with the use of ordered phase encoding, which retrospectively reorders the acquired signal with respect to its phase within the respiratory cycle. This technique is also referred to as respiratory compensation. The implementation of spatial saturation pulses reduces signal within the blood vessels, thereby eliminating pulsatility artifacts emanating from vessels.

2.1.2   Inversion Recovery

An inversion recovery sequence consists of an initial 180°pulse followed by a regular SE acquisition. TI denotes the time separating the inversion 180° pulse and the 90° SE pulse. The preliminary 180° pulse, inverts the z-magnetization without creating a phase coherence in the xy-plane.

Inversion recovery sequences enhance the T1 contrast between various tissues. The TI between the initial 180° and the subsequent 90° pulse determines the amplitude of the free induction decay. By adjusting TI, the signal from various tissues with a short T1 relaxation time can be nulled. The appropriate TI for nulling of a particular tissue can be calculated based on the following formula: TI = 0.69 T1$_{tissue}$. To null the signal of fat a TI of about 150 ms should be chosen. This form of fat supression is more robust than frequency select fat saturation pulses, which can be sensitive to field inhomogeneities.

2.1.3   Fast (Turbo) Spin-Echo Sequences

Conventional SE imaging with rapid acquisition and relaxation enhancement (RARE) has become widely available under various terms such as "turbo" or "fast" spin-echo (FSE). Similarly as in conventional SE imaging, the signal in FSE sequences is rendered by a 180° rephasing of spins. In FSE an initial 90° pulse is followed by a "train" of 180° pulses, each of which produces a detectable spin-echo. The number of echos within one TR is defined as the echo train length (ETL), while the time between 180° pulses is referred to as echo spacing. Thus within one TR data for several k-lines is acquired. Their exact number is determined by the ETL. An ETL of 1 is equivalent to a conventional SE sequence – in each MR acquisition data for a single k-line is acquired. If the ETL corresponds to the number of phase encoding steps, only one 90° excitation is required to fill all of k-space for the reconstruction of a complete image. Hence this sequence design is referred to as single-shot FSE. The echo spacing time determines the length of the acquisition. Under any circumstances the minimum echo spacing time should be chosen. High-performance imaging systems provide an echo spacing as low as 5 ms. For other systems echo spacing ranges between 10 and 15 ms.

During the TR interval transverse relaxation occurs with the time constant T2. Each of the spin-echos thus decreases in amplitude by a factor of exp (–TE/T2). The spin-echo arising from the last 180° pulses within the echo train is therefore of considerably less amplitude than the first. This may induce blurring as the low amplitude k-lines acquired at the end of the acquisition determine spatial resolution. Degradation of image quality due to blurring may be overcome by increasing the number of averaged excitations. For comparable image quality the number of averaged excitations for FSE sequences should be about twice that used for conventional SE imaging.

For most applications the ETL ranges between 4 and 16. Generally a large ETL results in shorter imaging times at the cost of fewer sections per acquisition and more blurring (Low et al. 1994). A short ETL, on the other hand, induces less blurring at the cost of longer imaging times. The length of the echo train defines both the minimum repetition time and image contrast. A short ETL permits the use of a shorter TR, thus assuring sufficient T1-weighting. Use of a long TR associated with a long ETL is void of residual T1 contrast and thereby automatically provides inherent T2-weighting. The TR used for T2-weighted FSE imaging usually ranges between 3000 and 5000 ms, exceeding that for conventional SE sequences. Effective echo times range between 95 and 110 ms for most applications. The effective echo time is always a multiple of the echo spacing.

Although used for both T1-weighted (Fig. 1) and T2-weighted (Fig. 2) imaging, the considerably greater time saving associated with T2-weighted FSE imaging has emphasized their use for many MR applications. For long ETL acquisitions the threshold set by the maximal length of a single breath-hold has been reached. The associated considerable reduction in motion artifacts has translated into better overall image quality. Compared to conventional SE acquisitions several differences do, however, exist (Fig. 2):

– The high frequency of 180° pulses creates the possibility of RF heating in the human body. While current levels are not critical, further reductions in the echo spacing may surpass allowable thresholds.
– FSE sequences are characterized by lower signal-to-noise ratios (SNR) and by greater blurring than conventional SE acquisitions. Increasing the number of averaged excitations can compensate for these differences.

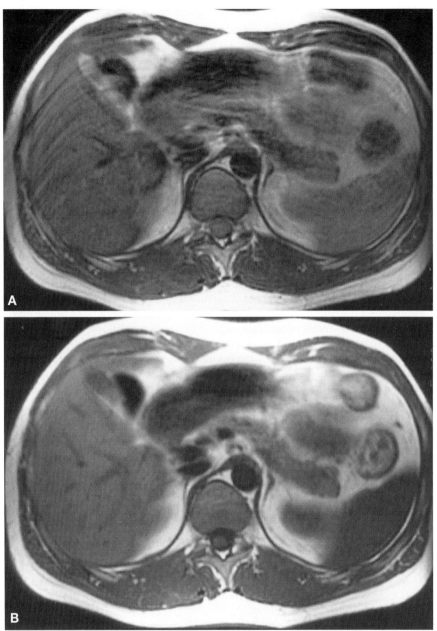

Fig. 1A, B. Comparison of T1-weighted conventional and fast SE sequences. (**A**) Despite the use of respiratory compensation algorithms, motion causes blurring in the non-breathheld conventional SE acquisition (TR/TE 300/9 ms, 4 NEX, acquisition time 4:49 min). (**B**) Blurring is reduced with breathheld FSE (TR/TE 300/14 ms, 1 NEX, acquisition time 34 s). Compared to conventional SE, FSE reduces imaging time considerably, permitting data acquisition in apnea. T1 contrast is sufficient in the FSE sequence

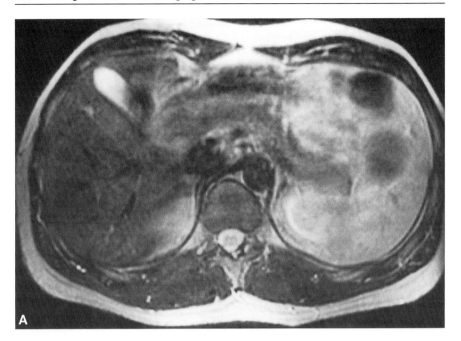

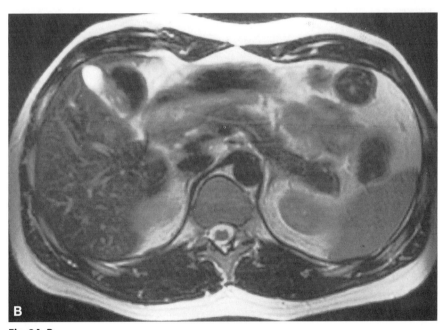

Fig. 2A, B

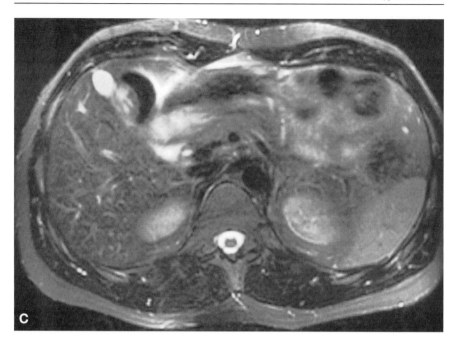

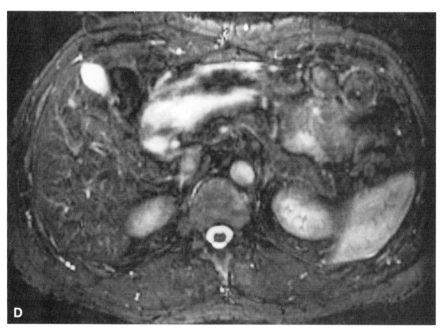

Fig. 2C, D

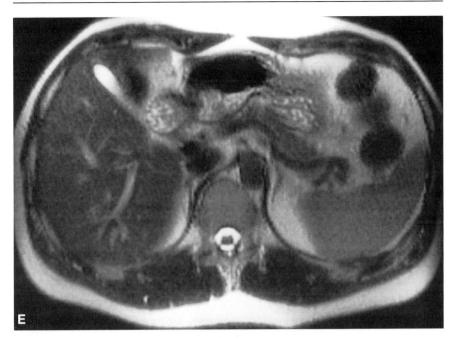

Fig. 2A–E. Comparison of various T2-weighted SE sequences.

(**A**) Conventional SE TR/TE 2500/80 ms, respiratory compensation, 2 NEX, acquisition time 19:53 min: Despite the use of respiratory compensation, motion artifacts corrupt the image quality of conventional T2-weighted images. Particularly the pancreas is poorly delineated. Signal from fat in the perirenal region can easily be distinguished from signal of fluid within the spinal canal. There is virtually no flow-related enhancement.

(**B**) FSE TR/TE 3750/108 ms, respiratory triggering, echo train length 12, 4 NEX, acquisition time 3:55 min: The availability of respiratory triggering in conjunction with shorter data acquisition times for FSE imaging considerably reduces motion artifacts. The pancreas can be delineated and even the pancreatic duct is easily identified. The signal intensity of fat as seen in the perirenal region is significantly higher than with conventional SE and at least visually overlaps with signal of fluid as seen in the spinal canal. The FSE sequence is more sensitive to slow flow, as evidenced by increased signal in some of the hepatic vessels.

(**C**) FSE TR/TE 3750/108 ms, respiratory triggering, echo train length 12, fat saturation, 4 NEX, acquisition time 3:55 min: The contrast between fluid- containing structures such as the spinal canal or gall bladder and other tissues can be significantly enhanced by using fat saturation in conjunction with FSE. There is virtually no loss with regard to image quality. The pancreatic duct remains visible.

(**D**) FSE inversion recovery TR/TE 3750/36 ms, TI 150 ms, respiratory triggering, 4 NEX, acquisition time 3:38 min: On the inversion recovery FSE image, the signal from fat is suppressed by using a 180° inversion pulse with an inversion time of 150 ms. This technique can be used if frequency select fat saturation is inhomogeneous due to field inhomogeneities or Eddy currents.

(**E**) Single-shot half-Fourier SE TR/TE 11825/99 ms, 0.5 NEX, acquisition time 12 s. Breath-held acquisition of T2-weighted images is possible with the use of a single-shot (snapshot) FSE sequence, using short echo spacing. The images are heavily T2-weighted, as evidenced by the high signal intensity of fluid in the spinal canal. Lack of motion artifacts permits delineation of the pancreas as well as the left adrenal gland

- Due to J-coupling effects the signal of fat is brighter than that of conventional SE imaging. Pathological water-containing tissues may thus be masked. Fat saturation or short TI inversion techniques can be used to enhance the contrast between water-containing and surrounding tissues.
- FSE sequences are less sensitive to flow effects. Slowly flowing blood in small vessels therefore frequently appears bright. In the periphery of parenchymal organs vascular signal may even be confused with lesions.
- FSE sequences are generally acquired with only a single echo. Collection of a second data set with a shorter echo, as frequently seen in conventional SE imaging, would double the length of the imaging time.

2.1.4   Half-Fourier Acquisition Single-Shot Fast Spin-Echo Sequences

In an effort to further reduce acquisition times the half-Fourier acquisition single-shot FSE (HASTE) sequence has been popularized for imaging structures in the abdomen which have a long T2-relaxation time with heavy T2-weighting. The technique combines single-shot FSE with half-Fourier reconstruction techniques. In this case only half of the data along k_y is acquired (positive or negative Fourier lines). This results in a further reduction of imaging times, permitting the collection of several T2-weighted sections during a single breath-hold. While SNR is decreased by $1/\sqrt{2}$SNR compared to conventional SE, there is no loss in image resolution. Use of a very long TE and TR results in a high-intensity representation of fluid-filled structures. Selective display of the biliary tree and pancreatic duct provides the basis for MR cholangio-pancreatography (MRCP). Similarly, the technique has been used in the assessment of the urinary tract. Lack of motion artifacts due to the underlying breath-held data acquisition have propelled these techniques into clinical imaging protocols of the abdomen and pelvis.

2.1.5   Fast Inversion Recovery

The fast inversion recovery SE (IRFSE) pulse sequence design combines a 180° inversion pulse with a FSE acquisition. The technique provides high-quality fat-saturated images. Since imaging time is lengthened, reflecting the incorporation of the inversion time, their use in the abdomen is generally limited to those cases in which frequency select fat saturation is insufficient (Constable et al. 1992).

The technique's sensitivity to water results in a 40% higher contrast-to-noise (CNR) of malignant liver lesions compared to FSE images, raising the sensitivity with regard to the detection of malignant liver lesions to 91.5% compared to 83.9% with FSE imaging (Kreft et al. 1995).

2.1.6   3D FSE Imaging

FSE imaging data can be acquired using a 3D Fourier transform. The 2D slice-selecting pulse is replaced by a pulse covering the entire volume of interest. The acquisition of overlapping signals in 3D volume imaging provides the basis for the reconstruction of contiguous sections as thin as 1 mm, with sufficient SNR. These sections in the z-axis permit multiplanar reconstructions. In their current implementation 3D FSE sequences remain vulnerable to motion artifacts. Their use in the evaluation of the biliary tract and the urinary system is currently under investigation.

2.2   Applications of Fast T2-Weighted Imaging

FSE acquisition strategies can be employed for the collection of both T1- and T2-weighted images of the abdomen. Less T1-weighting than in conventional SE or even T1-weighted GRE sequences coupled with only moderate savings in acquisition time have limited the use of T1-weighted FSE imaging in the abdomen. T2-weighted FSE imaging on the other hand has virtually replaced conventional T2-weighted SE sequences in the assessment of the abdominal organs. Substantial savings in data-acquisition times have reduced motion artifacts, contributing to vast improvements in overall image quality (Jung et al. 1996).

2.2.1   Liver

Reflecting the increased concentration of water, most benign and malignant focal hepatic lesions exhibit increased signal intensity (SI) on T2-weighted images. In many lesions the combined morphological appearance and SI on T2-weighted images may already be indicative of the nature of the lesion. Considerable overlap, however, exists regarding the differentiation between adenoma (Fig. 3), focal nodular hyperplasia, hepatocellular carcinoma (Fig. 4) metastases (Fig. 5) and hemangiomas (Fig. 6). Thus for characterization of focal hepatic lesions other sequences, including dynamic contrast-enhanced imaging, should be included in the imaging protocols.

FSE imaging has virtually replaced conventional T2-weighted SE in the assessment of the liver. The time gain associated with FSE imaging compared to conventional SE can be partially traded in for a longer TR to improve T2-weighting and a larger data matrix for better spatial resolution. Respiratory triggering of FSE sequences can further enhance image quality and diagnostic accuracy regarding the detection of focal liver lesions (Low et al. 1997).

Depending on system performance the acquisition time can be sufficiently shortened to acquire the T2-weighted images within a single breath-hold. The total absence of respiration-induced motion leads to a further improvement in image quality (Gaa et al. 1996; Van Hoe et al. 1996). Thus T2-weighted breath-hold imaging has been found to be more sensitive than conventional SE imaging,

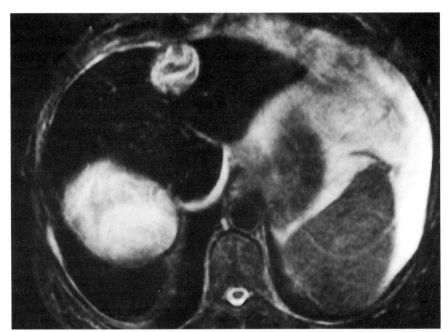

Fig. 3. Axial T2-weighted FSE image acquired with fat saturation demonstrates a blackened liver due to hemochromatosis in which two lesions are identified. Biopsy confirmed both lesions to be hepatic adenomas

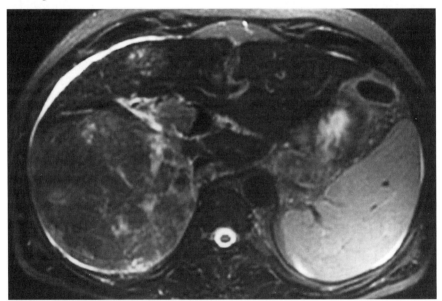

Fig. 4. Axial T2-weighted FSE image demonstrates a large hepatocellular carcinoma with portal venous infiltration replacing the entire right hepatic lobe. A small amount of ascites is present highlighting a mildly irregular contour of the liver

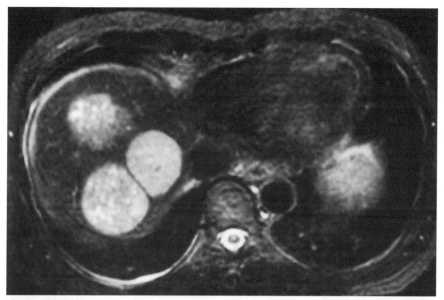

Fig. 5. Three hepatic metastases in a patient with colon carcinoma are identified in the dome of the liver on this axial T2 FSE image acquired with fat saturation. A small amount of ascites is present

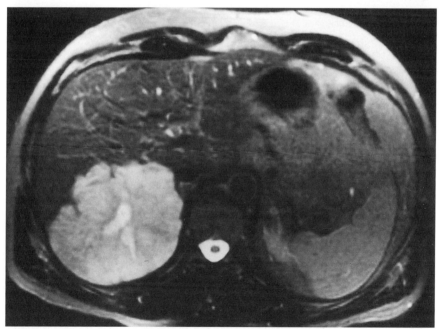

Fig. 6. Axial T2-weighted FSE image demonstrates a homogeneously bright mass in the right hepatic lobe. Mass morphology and SI are suggestive of a hemangioma, which in this case was confirmed surgically

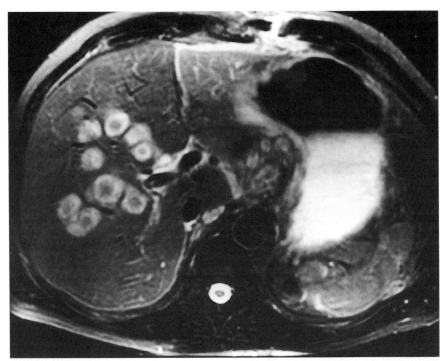

Fig. 7. Multiple cholangetic abscesses are seen on this T2-weighted FSE image acquired with fat saturation

regarding detection of liver masses, whilst imaging times are substantially reduced (Gaa et al. 1996).

A recent study has demonstrated that FSE T2-weighted images provide higher lesion-liver CNR and are preferred by readers to conventional SE T2-weighted imaging in terms of lesion detection (Schwartz et al. 1993; Low et al. 1993a,b). Furthermore, it has been demonstrated that the difference in SI ratios between benign and malignant is greater for FSE than for conventional SE images (Outwater et al. 1994). Recent results have also shown that the superior image quality in FSE imaging is sufficient to overcome even the disadvantage of not being capable of providing quantitative T2 relaxation data. Only in differentiating hypervascular metastases from hemangiomas (Figs. 5, 6) conventional SE images may be preferable (Schima et al. 1997).

The use of fat saturation with FSE can enhance lesion conspicuity (Fig. 7), particularly in fatty livers (Schwartz et al. 1993). Sensitivity in detection of focal malignant disease can be as high as 92%, compared to 89% without the use of fat saturation. Inversion recovery FSE sequences also provide excellent fat supression. In a recent comparison of four different breath-held T2-imaging strategies (Gaa et al. 1996) IR-FSE provided the highest liver-lesion CNR and was rated best with regard to image quality. IRFSE can also be used to differentiate focal fatty changes from benign or malignant focal mass lesions. While the signal of fat is nulled, lesions present with increased signal (Kane et al. 1993).

2.2.2 Pancreas

Unsurpassed soft tissue contrast, multiplanar imaging capabilities, and the ability to depict vascular structures without the use of contrast material have propelled MRI to the front-line of diagnostic imaging in the evaluation of upper abdominal symptoms. The assessment of the pancreas must be part of such an evaluation. Ideally, pancreatic disease should be ruled-in or ruled-out as a primary cause of the patient's symptomatology; furthermore, secondary involvement of the pancreas should be confirmed or excluded.

For maximal sensitivity T2-weighted sequences should be included in the assessment of the pancreas (Göhde et al. 1997). Conventional T2-weighted imaging has been limited by motion artifacts emanating from respiration and bowel peristalsis, pulsatility artifacts, and the inability to differentiate pancreatic tissue from heterogeneous surrounding structures. The introduction of FSE imaging has lessened these limitations to a considerable extent. The best image quality can be achieved using breath-held FSE strategies.

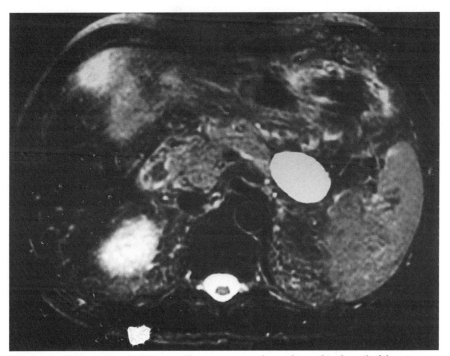

Fig. 8. Axial T2-weighted FSE image illustrates a pseudocyst located in the tail of the pancreas in a patient with pancreatitis

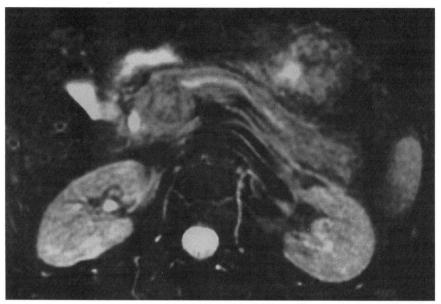

Fig. 9. Fat saturation in conjunction with T2-weighted FSE imaging is particularly helpful for depicting the pancreas. In this patient a mass identified in the head of the pancreas. The pancreatic duct is dilated in the corpus and tail of the pancreas

The main diagnostic focus of T2-weighted images in assessing pancreatic disease lies in the visualization of peripancreatic fluid or pseudocysts (Fig. 8) in pancreatitis. Associated complications such as bleeding, abscess formation or tissue necrosis can be characterized and quantified. Pancreatic duct dilatation or obstruction in malignant disease is also well depicted on T2-weighted FSE images. Increased SI is also associated with pancreatic carcinomas and metastases (Fig. 9), which have a longer T2 than normal pancreatic tissue, and especially of cystic or mucinous tumors (Outwater and Siegelman 1996). T2-weighted images have also been shown to be useful in the detection of insulinomas (Pavone et al. 1995).

2.2.3 Spleen

T2-weighted FSE imaging provides a comprehensive analysis of the slpeen, which generally exhibits a homogeneously high SI. The delineation of the spleen with respect to surrounding structures does not pose a problem. The size of the spleen is easily measured. Focal splenic lesions, such as cysts, hemangiomas, metastases or lymphoma, can be delineated as areas of increased SI.

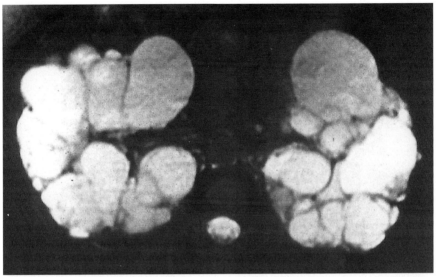

Fig. 10. Single-shot axial FSE image depicts the kidneys of an adult patient with polycystic kidney disease. The single-shot acquisition renders surrounding structures dark, highlighting the fluid filled cysts

2.2.4 Kidneys

Breath-held FSE imaging in the coronal plane provides a most comprehensive analysis of renal morphology and pathology. Both cysts and solid masses can be differentiated from normal renal parenchyma. Thus T2-weigthed FSE has been shown to be more sensitive than CT in the evaluation of focal renal lesions (Kreft et al. 1996). Fat saturation or the use of inversion recovery sequences can further enhance lesion conspicuity.

Cysts are characterized by a high homogeneous SI and the absence of a visible capsule (Fig. 10). Malignant renal or adrenal lesions, on the other hand, can present with increased or decreased SI on T2-weighted images relative to normal renal parenchyma (Fig. 11, 12).

In renal transplants T2-weighted images can depict post-operative complications including perional hematoms and lymphocedos. Delincation of artercal and venous vessels as well as assessment of parenchymal perfusion deficits requires use of contrast-enhanced fast gradient echo sequences.

2.2.5 MR Cholangio-pancreatography

MRCP became available with the implementation of fast and ultrafast imaging sequences. It is completely noninvasive, and does not require administration of contrast. MRCP is based on the hydrographic effect of bile fluids and sufficient suppression of surrounding structures (Figs. 13, 14). Ultrafast SE variants such as RARE

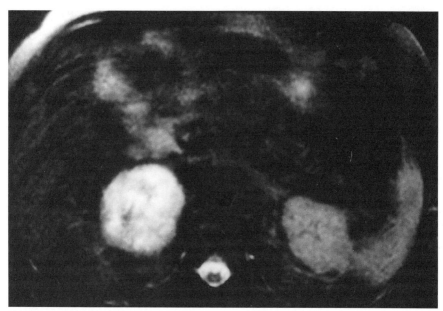

Fig. 11. Axial T2-weighted FSE image depicting a signal-intense mass in the upper pole of the right kidney. The increased signal suggests a nonadenomatous etiology. A primary renal carcinoma was confirmed at surgery

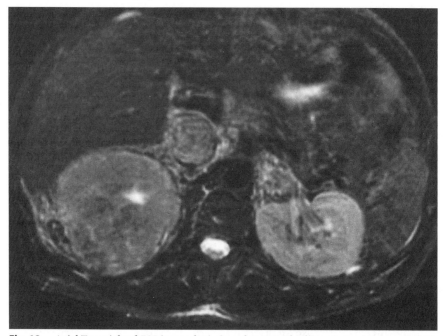

Fig. 12. Axial T2-weighted FSE image depicting a large renal cell carcinoma of the right kidney with high signal tumor thrombus propagating into the inferior vena cava

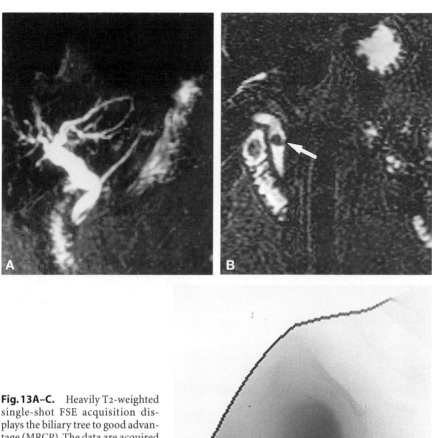

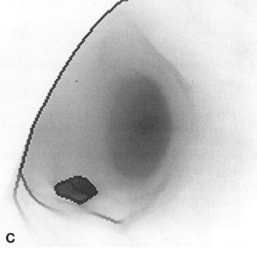

Fig. 13A–C. Heavily T2-weighted single-shot FSE acquisition displays the biliary tree to good advantage (MRCP). The data are acquired in a single breath-hold. (**A**) The MIP projection demonstrates moderate dilatation of the intrahepatic and extrahepatic biliary tree to the level of the papilla. (**B**) Analysis of the coronal individual images confirms the presence of the stone (*arrow*). (**C**) Virtual intraluminal endoscopic view from the papilla identifies the obstructing concrement

and HASTE allow T2-weighted snapshot imaging and effectively eliminate motion artifacts. The collection of all phase-encoding steps after a single excitation in 1.4 s allows motion artifacts to be avoided while SNRs remain sufficient. HASTE imaging proved to have a better SNR and CNR because of higher SI of bile compared to RARE imaging (Laubenberger et al. 1995) A possible drawback of turboSE or HASTE sequences using a high number of spin echoes is blurring in the phase-encoding direction. Because this blurring effect is more pronounced in tissues with shorter T2 relaxation times, this is not a limitation for MRCP. Therefore these snap-

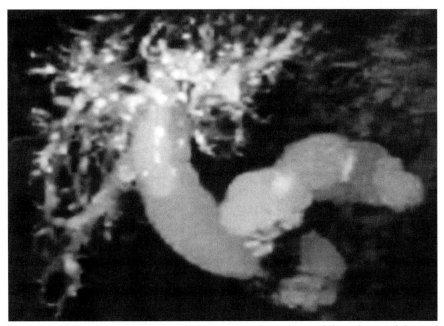

Fig. 14. MRCP sequence. Dilatation of intrahepatic and extrahepatic biliary ducts and the pancreatic duct by a confirmed neoplasia in the region of Vater's papilla. Maximum-intensity projection

shot sequences appear to be ideally suited for MRCP with reduced motion artifacts and acquisition times.

The heavily T2-weighted imaging sequence selectively depicts static or slowly flowing fluid with high SI (Fig. 13, 14). Fast-flowing liquids such as arterial, venous, or portal venous blood usually leave the acquisition volume between the initial radiofrequency (RF) pulse and the moment of readout procedure; these structures therefore are displayed with low signal intensities. This allows for the display of projectional images similar to ERCP. MRCP has been shown to be very accurate for the diagnosis of choledocholithiasis and biliary strictures. Biliary gas and flow voids may however result in false-positive findings (Wallner et al. 1991).

2.2.6 MR Pyeolgraphy

Images similar to those of conventional urography can be produced by the same heavily T2-weighted snapshot technique as employed for MRCP. Since no contrast agent needs to be administered, the technique is ideally suited for patients with renal insufficiency. Maximum-intensity projections provide a comprehensive 3D assessment of the morphology of the renal collecting system.

Compared to conventional urography, it can add important anatomical information by directly displaying structures near the urogenitary tract. MR pyelography can visualize urinary tract abnormalities and can provide additional information about renal parenchyma and the collecting system which might not be visible in conventional intravenous urography especially in patients with impaired renal function (Aerts et al. 1996).

Some authors describe limited visualization of normal, not dilated ureters with this sequence (Catalano et al. 1996). If a 3D sequence is performed in a non-breath-held manner, respiratory triggering and the administration of furosemide enhances image quality (Di-Girolamo et al. 1996). The use of negative bowel contrast agents eliminate image artifacts arising from high signal of intestinal fluids (Hirohashi et al. 1997).

3   Fast 2D Gradient-Echo Imaging

Fast 2D GRE acquisitions permit data collection in apnea. For patient comfort a breath-hold should be limited to 30 s. Breath-holding in end-inspiration is generally associated with good patient compliance. In abdominal MRI examinations breath-held 2D GRE techniques are employed for various reasons:
a) to provide an alternative to T1 weighted SE images,
b) to characterize the enhancement pattern of lesions within parenchymal organs in conjunction with the intravenous administration of paramagnetic contrast agents, and
c) to quantitate the contents of intracellular fat.

3.1   Technique Considerations

The implementation of ultrafast data-acquisition strategies has vastly reduced the minimum repetition and echo times used for gradient-echo imaging. GRE acquisitions now permit data collection in apnea. Imaging during suspended respiration, which for patient comfort should be limited to 30 s, eliminates respiratory artifacts and blurring caused by motion (Low et al. 1993a,b). Recent hardware and software improvements have resulted in progressively shorter repetition and echo times and thus in improved spatial resolution and/or increased coverage. State-of-the-art fast gradient-echo techniques provide imaging data covering the entire abdomen from diaphragm to the lower poles of the kidneys with contiguous 8-mm sections in the axial plane.

There are two different GRE data-acquisition strategies: sequential and multiplanar GRE.

3.1.1   Sequential GRE Acquisitions

GRE data is collected for a single section using a minimum repetition time prior to going on to the next section. This technique is referred to as fast GRE (GE Medical Systems) or turbo fast low-angle shot (Turbo-FLASH, Siemens Medical Systems). Repetition times between 7 and 10 ms allow images to be acquired at a rate of about 1/s.

3.1.2   Multiplanar GRE Acquisitions

This technique is referred to as fast multiplanar spoiled gradient-echo imaging (FMPSPGR, GE Medical Systems) or FLASH (Siemens Medical Systems). The use of a longer TR (100–150 ms) in conjunction with minimum TEs in addition to RF phase spoiling of the residual transverse magnetization assures T1 weighting. Use of the minimum TE furthermore leads to maximal coverage and spatial resolution.

As TR times are decreased, increased spin saturation reduces SNR and tissue contrast (Fig. 15). To obtain high SNR and high contrast on images while maintaining acquisition times sufficiently short for breath-hold imaging, an interleaved acquisition order can be used. The multiplanar interleaved version of this sequence acquires the same k-space view at various scan locations. The procedure is repeated until k-space views from all scan locations are acquired within the pass (Low et al. 1993a,b). The number of scan locations within the pass determines the number of slices per acquisition. The interval between successive RF excitation pulses at the same location is determined by the minimum TR multiplied by the number of slices.

Although images are still being acquired at the same rate, the effective repetition time is substantially increased. This allows higher RF flip angles to be used, increasing image SNR and providing better image contrast (Fig. 15). In addition, contiguous slices can be collected without slice cross-talk in a multiple-pass interleaved acquisition. Low et al. (1993a,b) have shown that the Ernst angle for such a multiplanar acquisition with a repetition time of around 150 ms ranges between 50° and 60°. The effective repetition time (100–150 ms) should be chosen on the basis of the patients' ability to perform breath-holding and the number of sections needed to cover the area of interest (Fig. 15). Lower repetition times should be combined with slightly lower flip angles. Semelka et al. (1991) showed that multiplanar GRE provides a significantly higher SNR than sequential GRE imaging (Fig 15).

3.2   T1-Weighted GRE Imaging

T1-weighted sequences have been shown to be important for tissue characterization in the liver and in other abdominal organs. Short TR/TE SE sequences, acquired over several minutes have been most frequently employed to achieve T1 weighting. With fast 2D GRE sequence designs a similar number of images can be collected within a comfortable breath-hold (Semelka et al. 1991; Fig. 15).

The contrast in GRE sequences depends on a large number of factors, including field strength and imaging parameters. At 1.5-T field strength T1 weighting of 2D GRE sequences is achieved by combining the minimum TR with a minimum TE and a relatively high flip angle (60°–90°; Saini and Nelson 1995; Semelka et al. 1991). Additional T1 weighting can be achieved by using gradient or RF spoiling of residual transverse magnetization (see Chap. 1). At the cost of slightly prolonging imaging times, excellent T1 weighting can also be achieved by employing section-selective magnetization-prepared (MP) pulses (de Lange et al. 1996).

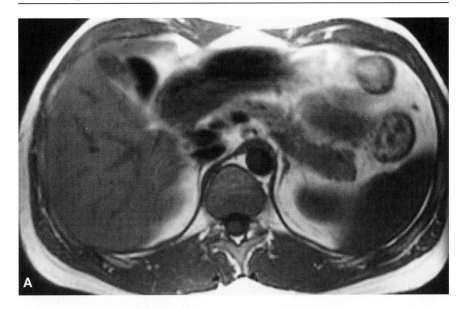

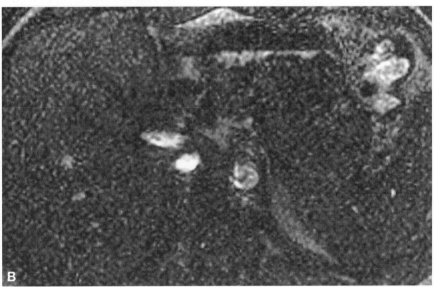

Fig. 15A, B.   Three T1-weighted GRE sequences in comparison to T1-weighted conventional SE:
(**A**) Conventional SE image TR/TE 300/9 ms, 4 NEX, acquisition time 4:49 min displays excellent
T1 contrast. Respiratory motion causes blurring which limits the ability to delineate the pancreas.
(**B**) Sequentially acquired GRE image TR/TE 7/1.6 ms, 1 NEX, acquisition time 1.6 s. Flow-related
enhancement is evidenced by bright signal in the inferior vena cava and the portal vein as well
as the aorta. The images are acquired breath-held, thereby eliminating respiratory motion artifacts. The very short repetition time reduces the signal-to-noise ratio compared to the conventional SE image.

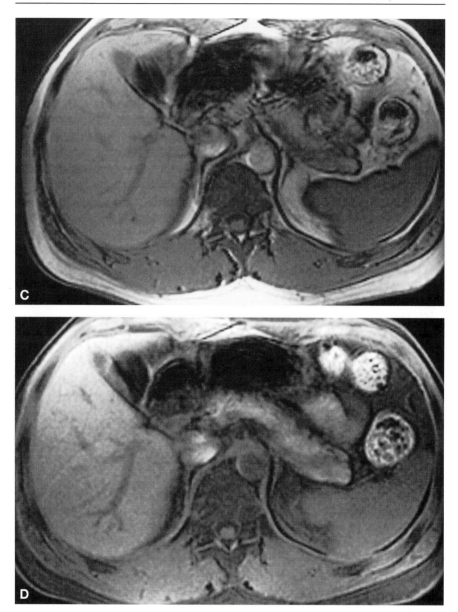

Fig. 15C, D

(C) Multiplanar spoiled GRE images TR/TE 150/1.6 ms, 1 NEX, acquisition time 26 s. The acquisition time of 26 s permits the collection of 20 contiguous images. Excellent image quality is related to the breath-held data acquisition. The longer TR provides improved signal-to-noise ratio. Excellent T1 weighting is illustrated by the contrast difference between the liver and the spleen.

(D) The multiplanar spoiled GRE sequence can be acquired with fat saturation. Fat saturation has been found to be particularly useful for analysis of the pancreas, which in this image is easily delineated from surrounding structures

A 180° MP pulse separated from the beginning of the GRE sequence by a delay time of 200 ms should be used in conjunction with the minimal repetition and echo times and a low flip angle of 10° (de Lange et al. 1996).

In the abdomen the degree of T1 weighting can be assessed based on the spleen-liver signal-difference-to-noise (S-D/N) value. Compared to conventional short TR/TE SE imaging, both sequential and multiplanar GRE imaging have been found to have better T1 weighting as evidenced by a greater spleen-liver S-D/N value (Semelka et al. 1991). The same study demonstrated the multiplanar mode to be superior to sequentially acquired GRE images with regard to SNR, overall image quality, and S-D/N values (Semelka et al. 1991). Similar results were reported by Taupitz et al. (1992), who also illustrated the superiority of multiplanar gradient-echo imaging with regard to signal and contrast characteristics over conventional short TR/TE SE imaging. Based on these findings, breath-held multiplanar GRE sequences should be used in the abdomen for T1-weighted imaging.

3.3   Dynamic Contrast-Enhanced GRE Imaging

Excellent inherent T1 contrast, absence of respiratory artifacts, extended anatomical coverage, and sufficient temporal resolution make multiplanar 2D spoiled GRE sequences well suited for the dynamic display of intraparenchymal signal changes following the intravenous bolus administration of T1-shortening paramagnetic gadolinium chelates. Assessment of parenchymal enhancement has been shown to augment the diagnostic yield of an MR examination with regard to both lesion detection and, even more significantly, lesion characterization. Ensuing increases in diagnostic accuracy thus reflect both improved sensitivity and specificity (Saini and Nelsion 1995; Low et al. 1993a,b; de Lange et al. 1996; Eilenberg et al. 1990; Rofsky et al. 1991; Semelka et al. 1992a,b, 1993a,b, 1994; Mathieu et al. 1991; Hamm et al. 1994; Whitney et al. 1993; Peterson et al. 1996; Ramani et al. 1997; Göhde et al. 1997). Most investigators have proposed the use of a multiplanar sequence to exploit higher SNRs (Fig. 15). These sequences are referred to either as FMPSPGR or FLASH.

To achieve optimal results the contrast should be administered as a tight bolus either by hand or by power injector (3 ml/s) followed by a generous saline flush (20–40 ml). To permit full analysis of the contrast dynamics, images of the entire organ need to be obtained during several phases of enhancement: prior to the administration of contrast material, during the arterial phase at 20 s, during the portal venous phase at 50–100 s, and during the equilibrium phase 3–5 min after beginning the intravenous administration of contrast material (Saini and Nelson 1995; Fig. 16). For improved organ delineation and lesion conspicuity in the pancreas and liver the signal of fat can be suppressed by either employing frequency selective fat saturation pulses or choosing the length of the TE to coincide with the time when fat and water are out of phase (Saini and Nelson 1995).

Based on the administration of contrast, cysts can generally be distinguished from solid masses regardless of their location. Beyond this there are pathognomonic enhancement profiles permitting the characterization of focal lesions in various parenchymal organs.

3.3.1 Liver

Dynamic contrast-enhanced GRE imaging has been shown to be useful in the assessment of the liver (Peterson et al. 1996; Yamashita et al. 1996; Hamm et al. 1994; Semelka et al. 1994; Whitney et al. 1993; Mathieu et al. 1991). The dual blood supply to the liver via the hepatic artery and the portal vein provides an oppor-

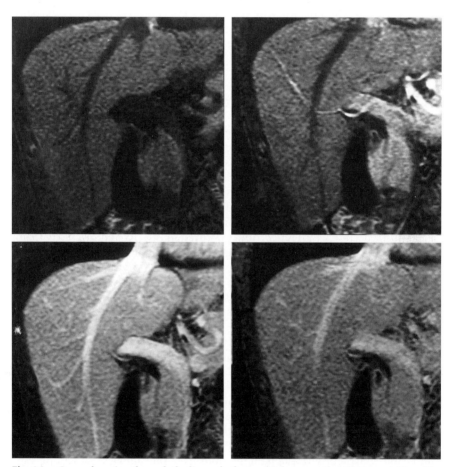

Fig. 16. Coronal section through the liver of a fast multiplanar spoiled GRE acquisition. The first phase was acquired prior to the administration of intravenous contrast material. The second image set corresponds to the arterial phase, the third to the portal venous phase, and the fourth to the equilibrium phase acquired 3–4 minutes following intravenous administration of paramagnetic contrast. The dynamic enhancement of arteries, veins, and hepatic parenchyma can be observed

tunity to maximize diagnostic accuracy by collecting several image sets during the various vascular phases. The images are generally acquired in the axial plane. For assessment of lesions located in the dome of the liver, or analysis of the hepatic vasculature (Fig. 16) the coronal or sagittal plane may be used. Pulsatility artifacts emanating from the heart may on occasion complicate interpretation of coronal GRE images, particularly those collected in the arterial phase immediately following the intravenous administration of paramagnetic contrast.

Dynamic GRE imaging has been shown to enhance sensitivity, particularly regarding the detection of small hepatocellular carcinomas in patients with chronic liver damage (Peterson et al. 1996; Yamashita et al. 1996). In fact, multiphase dynamic MRI was shown to be superior to helical CT for hepatocellular carcinomas (Yamashita et al. 1996) and to conventional T1- and T2-weighted imaging in the detection of metastases (Peterson et al. 1996).

Beyond enhancing sensitivity, dynamic contrast-enhanced 2D GRE imaging permits characterization of hepatic lesions, thereby increasing the specificity of hepatic MRI. A prospective blinded study of 55 patients with benign and 52 patients with

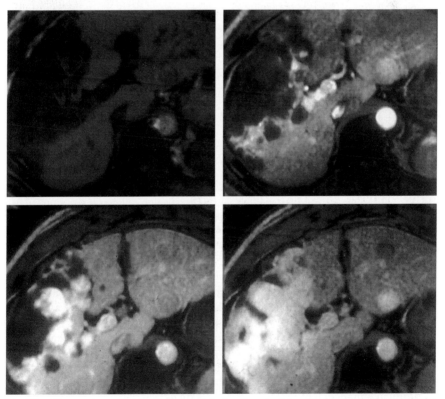

Fig. 17. Hemangioma depicted before and during the arterial, venous, and equilibrium phases following the intravenous administration of paramagnetic contrast on an axial fast multiplanar spoiled GRE acquisition. The nodular centripetal enhancement is pathognomonic for the diagnosis of hemangioma

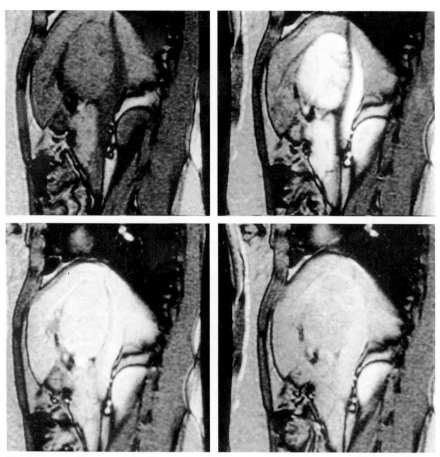

Fig. 18. FNH illustrated on a fast multiplanar GRE acquisition with image sets acquired before and during the arterial, portal venous, and equilibrium phases following the administration of intravenous contrast material. The characteristically homogeneous enhancement during the arterial phase followed by early wash-out is pathognomonic for the diagnosis of FNH. The sagittal plane is well suited for depicting masses affecting the dome of the liver

malignant focal liver lesions showed dynamic contrast-enhanced fast GRE imaging to add significant information to nonenhanced MR studies. Distinction between benign and malignant lesions was facilitated. There are in fact two benign lesions which can be identified as such based on their virtually pathognomonic enhancement profile: hemangioma and focal nodular hyperplasia (FNH).

Cavernous hemangiomas are the most common tumors of the liver (Fig. 17). Semelka et al. (1994) described three enhancement patterns for hemangiomas:
a) uniform enhancement during the arterial phase;
b) peripheral nodular enhancement progressing centripetally to uniform enhancement, and
c) peripheral nodular enhancement with persistent hypointensity centrally.

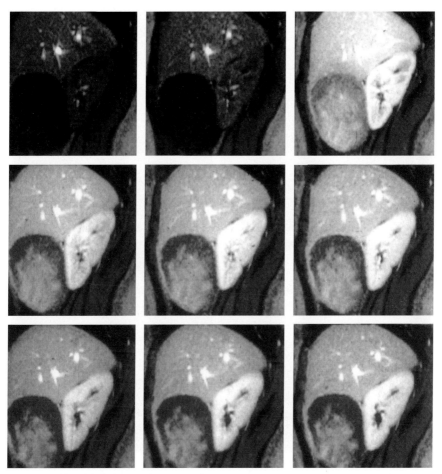

Fig. 19. Hepatic adenoma displayed on multiple phases of a sequentially acquired fast GRE acquisition. The images display the mass before and during various phases following the intravenous administration of paramagnetic contrast material. The enhancement pattern is unlike that seen in hemangiomas or focal nodular hyperplasia. Based upon MR findings, a hepatic adenoma cannot be differentiated from hepatocellular carcinoma

The enhancement pattern appears related to the size of the lesion: while uniform, early enhancement is most commonly seen in small lesions (< 1.5 cm), persistent central areas of hypointensity are generally associated with large lesions (> 5 cm; Fig. 17) Whitney et al.(1993) showed contrast-enhanced multiplanar spoiled GRE imaging to be significantly more accurate in characterizing hemangiomas than T2-weighted imaging. Hemangiomas were diagnosed with 100% specificity and 95% accuracy, based on a pathognomonic nodular, globular enhancement pattern, with progressive centripetal filling-in. Malignancies, on the other hand, demonstrated hypo- or hyperintense enhancement relative to

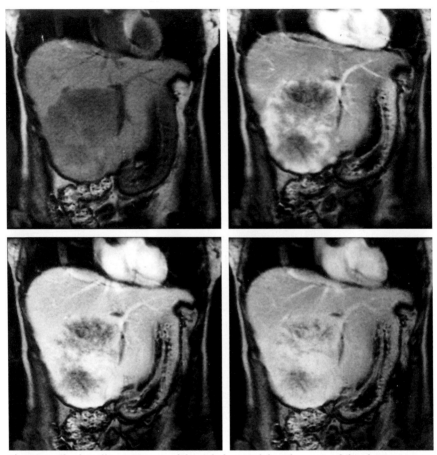

Fig. 20. Fibrolamellar carcinoma of the right hepatic lobe. The mass exhibits heterogeneous enhancement in the arterial, portal, and equilibrium phases following the administration of paramagnetic contrast, as shown on these fast multiplanar GRE images. Based on its enhancement profile, the diagnosis of fibrolamellar carcinoma can be suspected. Definitive differentiation from other primary or secondary malignant lesions of the liver is not possible

liver, often with a hyperintense peripheral progressively centripetal pattern. However, no malignancy displayed a nodular enhancement pattern.

FNH of the liver is characterized by a completely different, albeit similarly pathognomonic enhancement pattern. FNH is frequently found in adult women, although 10%–20% occur in men. The origin of FNH is unknown, but a vascular malformation is suspected. Although a subject of continued speculation and discussion, the tumor genesis appears to be unrelated to the use of birth control pills. FNH contains hepatocytes, Kupffer cells, and fibrous tissue. A frequently seen central scar is made up of venoles and small bile ducts surrounded by fibrous tissue. The lesion is generally of low SI on T1-weighted images and mildly

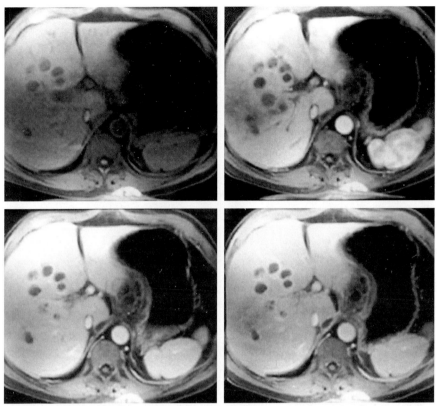

Fig. 21. Multiple cholangetic abscesses displayed to good advantage on the dynamic contrast enhanced fast multiplanar GRE acquisition. The lesions demonstrate rim enhancement on the equilibrium phase images

increased SI on T2-weighted images. The mainly arterial supply of the lesion is reflected by very early and homogeneous enhancement followed by rapid wash-out and equilibration with the surrounding hepatic parenchyma (Fig. 18). Accordingly, on equilibrium images, FNH lesions are frequently indistinguishable from surrounding hepatic tissue (Fig. 18). Only the centrally located scar, which is generally hyperintense on T2-weighted images, demonstrates late enhancement on the equilibrium phase images.

A study of 25 patients with FNH showed the characteristic early arterial enhancement on dynamic 2D GRE images in all lesions, while enhancement within the scar on equilibrium images was demonstrated in only 10 of the 25 tumors (Mathieu et al. 1991). In a different study FNH was diagnosed more often and with a higher degree of confidence on the basis of dynamic contrast-enhanced GRE sequences than nonenhanced sequences (Hamm et al. 1994). Correct timing of the arterial phase data acquisition is crucial for a confident diagnosis of FNH.

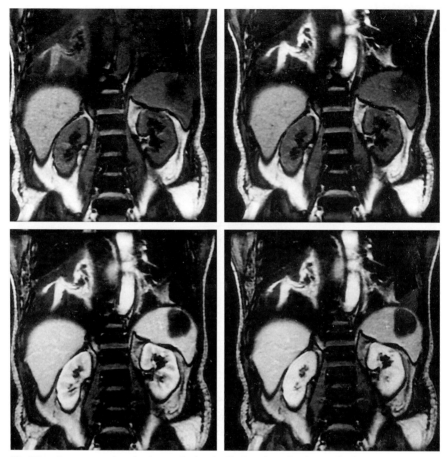

Fig. 22. Posttraumatic splenic cyst is clearly displayed on the fast multiplanar GRE acquisition acquired before and during the arterial, portal venous, and equilibrium phases following the injection of paramagnetic contrast

Other lesions, including hepatic adenoma (Fig. 19) or hepatocellular carcinoma (Fig. 20) cannot be distinguished from oneanother based on their enhancement patterns. Based on distribution as well their characteristic wall enhancement abscesses may be recognized as such on the dynamic contrast-enhanced images (Fig. 21).

3.3.2 Spleen

Dynamic contrast-enhanced 2D GRE imaging has been shown to improve lesion conspicuity and detectability over conventional T1- and T2-weighted SE sequences (Ramani et al. 1997; Mirowitz et al. 1991). Similar to the liver, the spleen is best imaged in the axial plane. Care must be taken not to misinterpret the heterogeneous appearance of the spleen in the first minute following contrast admin-

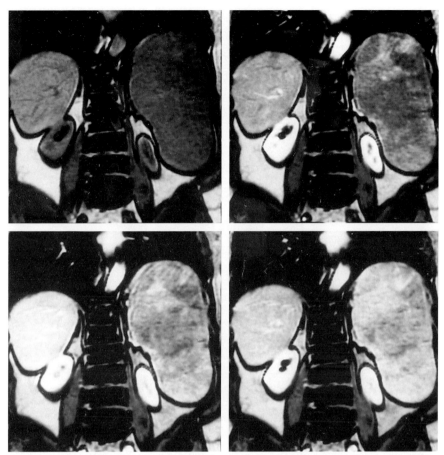

Fig. 23. Splenic lymphoma is the cause of persistently heterogeneous enhancement of the spleen following the intravenous administration of paramagnetic contrast. Heterogeneous enhancement is normal on arterial phase images. Persistent heterogeneity into the portal venous and equilibrium phases, as seen in this case, must be considered abnormal

istration, which has been shown to occur regularly with or without portal hypertension (Mirowitz et al. 1991).

Splenic cysts are easily identified as such on the dynamically acquired images (Fig. 22). Hemangiomas of the spleen reveal enhancement patterns similar to those described for hepatic hemangiomas. Since these features have been shown reliably to distinguish hemangiomas from other benign and malignant liver lesions, it may be reasonable to consider that lesions in the spleen demonstrating nodular peripheral contrast enhancement with progressive filling-in do indeed also represent hemangiomas (Ramani et al. 1997). No pathognomonic enhancement features have been reported for hamartomas or other focal splenic masses (Ramani et al. 1997). Persistent heterogeneity on the late-phase equilib-

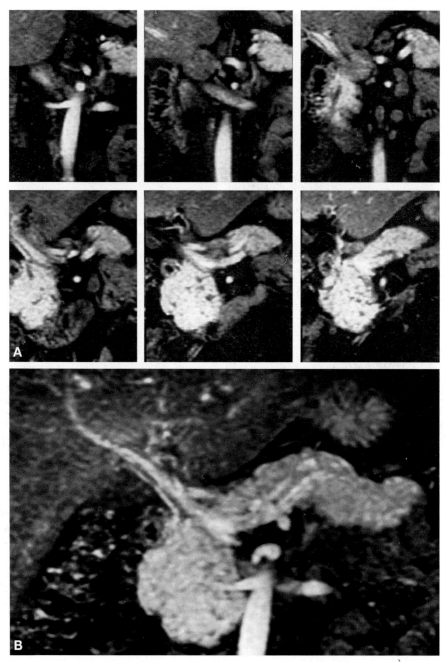

Fig. 24A, B. Six contiguous 8-mm sections of a fast multiplanar spoiled GRE acquisition, collected in the early arterial phase following the administration of paramagnetic contrast (**A**) can be combined into a single maximum-intensity projection image (**B**) delineating the contours of the pancreas to good advantage

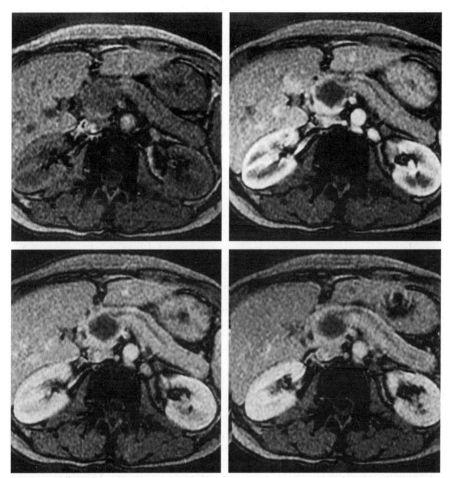

Fig. 25. Pancreatic carcinoma located in the pancreatic head depicted on fast multiplanar GRE images acquired before and during the arterial, portal venous, and equilibrium phases following the administration of paramagnetic contrast. Dilatation of the pancreatic duct becomes apparent on the contrast-enhanced images. The pancreas is best delineated in the early arterial phase images

rium images should trigger associations with diffusely infiltrating processes such as leukemia or lymphoma (Fig. 23).

3.3.3 Pancreas

More than any other organ in the abdomen, depiction of the pancreas has been limited by motion artifacts induced by respiration, peristalsis and pulsatility as well as the inability to differentiate pancreatic tissue from heterogeneous

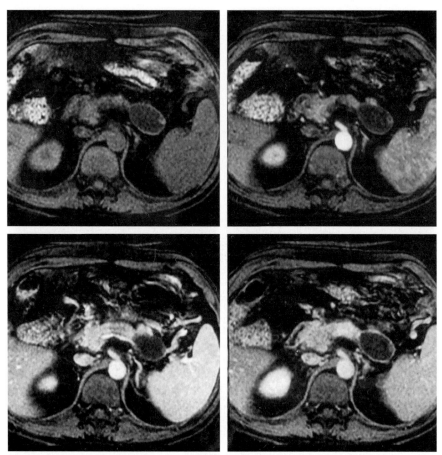

Fig. 26. Pseudocyst originating from the tail of the pancreas following a bout of pancreatitis. The lesion is well delineated on the fast multiplanar GRE images. Breath-held data acquisition assures maximal image quality without corruption by respiratory motion. Massive dilatation of the intra- and extrahepatic biliary tree and the pancreatic duct is evident on these fast multiplanar GRE images acquired before and during arterial, portal venous, and equilibrium phases following the administration of paramagnetic contrast

surrounding structures. In addition to the acquisition of standard T1- and T2-weighted sequences, most authors agree on the need for fat-supressed contrast-enhanced T1-weighted sequences (Hagspiel et al. 1994; Mitchell et al. 1992b). Dynamic, multiplanar gradient-echo imaging permits the simultaneous assessment of the entire upper abdomen, including the pancreas during the peak SI phase (Göhde et al. 1997; Hamed et al. 1992; Fig. 24).

A recent study assessing the performance of various sequences in 101 consecutive patients for evaluation of the pancreas found that the contrast-enhanced fast multiplanar spoiled GRE sequence performed better than conventional SE MRI (Göhde et al. 1997; Figs. 25–27). This study confirmed the unequivocal supe-

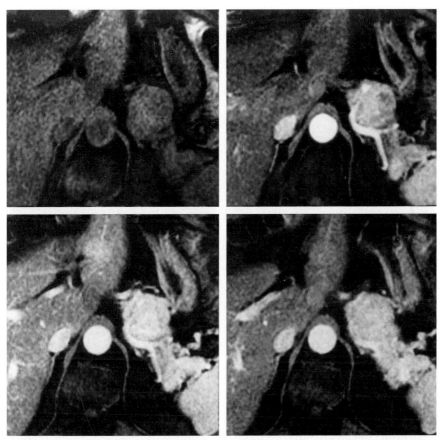

Fig. 27. A mass identified in the corpus of the pancreas exhibits homogeneous enhancement in the arterial phase on these contrast-enhanced multiplanar GRE images. The early arterial enhancement is suggestive of an endocrine tumor. In this case an insulinoma was confirmed

riority of breath-held, contrast-enhanced fast GRE imaging over conventional SE sequences in the analysis of the pancreas. Taking advantage of the strong enhancement of the pancreatic tissue during the first-pass distribution of the paramagnetic agent, which has been shown to reach a maximum at 40 s following intravenous bolus administration (Sittek et al. 1995), the pancreatic morphology is best delineated on the early dynamic GRE image set (Figs. 25–27). CNRs were highest for the arterial phase images.

Assessment of readers' diagnostic accuracy and confidence regarding the detection of pancreatic pathology was found to reflect directly the ability to delineate the pancreatic tissue itself. Regarding the detection of pancreatic pathology, the sensitivity and specificity of dynamic GRE imaging (87% and 100%) compared favorably with those of T1-weighted SE (sensitivity: 50%; specificity: 96%), fat supressed T2-weighted SE (sensitivity: 60%; specificity: 93%) and contrast-enhanced T1-weighted SE imaging with fat saturation (sensitivity: 53%;

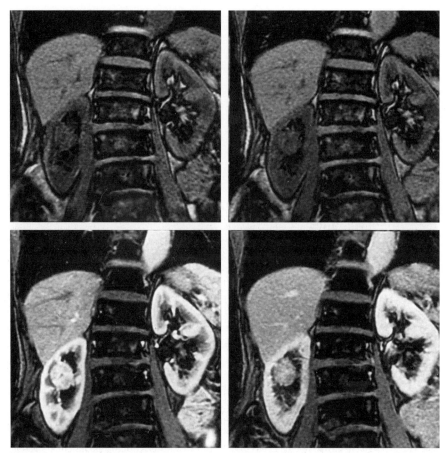

Fig. 28. Homogeneously enhancing round mass identified in the middle portion of the right kidney on fast multiplanar GRE images acquired before and during the arterial, venous, and equilibrium phases following the administration of contrast. The homogeneous enhancement and round morphology are suggestive of an oncocytoma, which in this case was confirmed intraoperatively

specificity: 90%). Analysis of receiver operator characteristics confirmed the superior diagnostic performance of the dynamic contrast-enhanced sequence (Göhde et al. 1997).

For optimal diagnostic accuracy, dynamic GRE imaging of the pancreas should be performed in the axial plane rather than the coronal plane. Furthermore, the use of fat saturation is helpful as it enhances the contrast of the pancreas relative to surrounding structures (Göhde et al. 1997; Fig. 24).

With optimal technique pancreatic cysts (Fig. 26) can easily be differentiated from solid masses (Figs. 25, 27). Carcinomatous lesions are generally characterized by reduced enhancement in the early arterial phase. Islet cell tumors, on the other hand, generally exhibit avid homogeneous early arterial enhancement

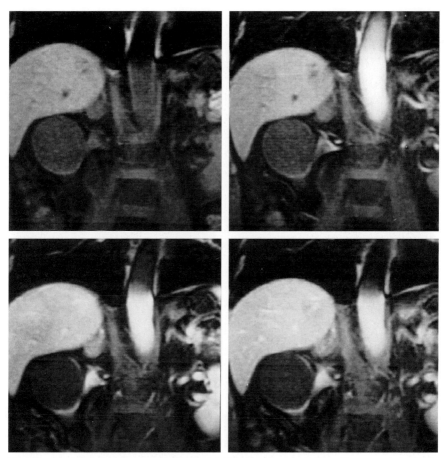

Fig. 29. Cystc mass of the upper pole of the right kidney demonstrates enhancement of a thickened rim on the dynamically acquired fast multiplanar GRE images. A renal cell carcinoma in the thickened wall was confirmed intraoperatively

(Fig. 27). Dynamic contrast-enhanced GRE imaging has in fact been shown to be more accurate in the detection of islet cell tumors than spiral CT (Semelka et al. 1993a).

3.3.4 Kidneys

On dynamic contrast-enhanced GRE images the kidneys are displayed to best advantage in the coronal plane (Figs. 28–32). Contrast-enhanced dynamic gradient-echo imaging of the kidneys has been shown to be useful in both detecting and characterizing simple renal cysts and solid neoplasms (Eilenberg et al. 1990; Rofsky et al. 1991; Semelka et al. 1992b, 1993b; Figs. 28–31).

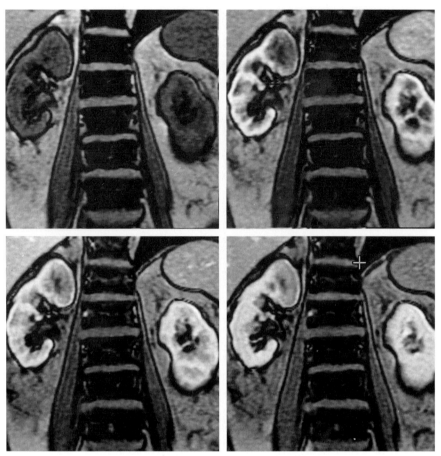

Fig. 30. Renal mass seen on fast multiplanar GRE images acquired before and during the arterial, venous, and equilibrium phases following the administration of paramagnetic contrast. The mass is characterized by heterogeneous enhancement and was confirmed to be a renal cell carcinoma

The administration of paramagnetic contrast is safe, with a low incidence of anaphylactoid reactions. In addition, there are no nephrotoxic effects even in patients with impaired renal function. Eilenberg et al. (1990) reported on three distinct enhancement patterns of renal cell carcinoma:
a) irregular peripheral enhancement with only minimal heterogeneous central enhancement,
b) heterogeneous enhancement, and
c) mild homogeneous enhancement (Figs. 29–31).

Further characterization of solid masses as benign or malignant lesions has not been possible. Only the characteristic round shape and homogeneous enhance-

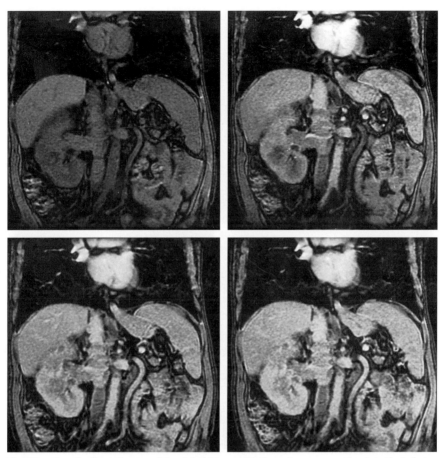

Fig. 31. Renal cell carcinoma of the right kidney with thrombus propagating into the inferior vena cava is displayed on these fast multiplanar GRE images acquired before and during the arterial, venous, and equilibrium phases following the administration of paramagnetic contrast. Enhancement of the thrombus in the inferior vena cava is indicative of the presence of tumor thrombus, which was confirmed intraoperatively

ment of most oncocytomas may be suggestive of the correct histological typing (Fig. 28). Evidence of fat on the precontrast GRE images suggests an angiomyolipoma.

Propagation of thrombus into the renal veins and inferior vena cava is also well seen on breath-held contrast-enhanced fast GRE images. Enhancement of the thrombus confirms the presence of tumor tissue within the thrombotic material (Fig. 31). Lack of enhancement is indicative of a benign etiology (Fig. 32)

Paramagnetic contrast is excreted rapidly into the renal collecting system. Acquisition of a delayed set of multiplanar gradient-echo images in the coronal plane often illustrates the presence of contrast material in the renal calices and proximal ureters.

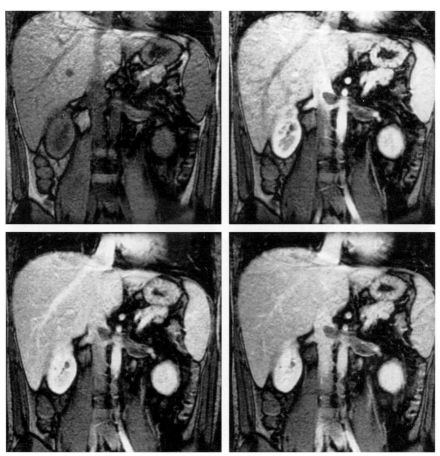

Fig. 32. Coronal fast multiplanar GRE images demonstrate thrombus in the left renal vein. A lack of enhancement within the thrombus is indicative of a bland etiology

3.4   Phase-Shift Gradient-Echo Imaging

At 1.5-T (64 MHz) field strength lipid and water spins have a frequency difference of about 224 Hz. Thus a phase cycling of water and lipid spins occurs every 2.24 ms following the excitation pulse. At this interval lipid and water spins are alternatively in and out of phase. Thus an echo time of 2.2–2.3 ms renders fat and water protons "out of phase," while an echo time of 4.2 ms renders them "in phase." Various paramaters have been used to acquire in- and out-of-phase GRE images. Among the many evaluated techniques, fast, multiplanar, spoiled, breath-held GRE imaging with a TR of 100–150 ms, a flip angle of 60° and a receiver bandwith of ± 32 kHz appears most promising. For out-of-phase imaging a TE of 2.3 ms is used and for in-phase imaging 4.6 ms. If the minimum achievable TE exceeds 2.3 ms, a TE of 6.9 ms is chosen for out-of-phase imaging. To allow breath-held data acquisition only one signal can be averaged. Tsushima et al. (1993) point out that it is important to acquire the in- and out-of-phase images with the same transmit of power and receiver gain settings. This can be achieved if the sequences are acquired following tuning at an echo time which lies between the two chosen echo times for the in- and out-of-phase images.

The SI of the opposed phase images depends on the proportion of lipid and water content within the tissue. In contrast to nonlipid containing tissue, whose SI remains identical on the in- and out-of-phase images, fat-containing tissue is characterized by a precipitous decrease in SI on the opposed phase images (Korobkin et al. 1995; Bilbey et al. 1995; Tsushima et al. 1993; Mitchell et al. 1992a). This effect can be exploited in various manners. With in- and out-of-phase GRE imaging the liver can be assessed for fatty infiltration. The latter is confirmed if a signal difference between the two image sets can be ascertained (Saini and Nelson 1995).

In- and out-of-phase GRE imaging has also been advocated for characterizing adrenal mass lesions (Figs. 33–35). The lipid contents within a particular adrenal lesion can be quantitated using an SI index based on SI measurements of the lesion in in-phase and opposed-phase GRE images (Tsushima et al. 1993): SI index = [(SI on IP–SI on OP)/(SI on IP)] × 100%, where IP stands for in-phase and OP for out-of-phase. Some investigators have proposed expressing the SI index relative to other reference tissues such as liver or muscle (Korobkin et al. 1995; Bilbey et al. 1995).

The use of chemical shift imaging as a differentiating parameter is predicated upon the well-known fact that adrenal adenomas contain a large amount of cytoplasmic lipid (Fig. 33), in contrast to adrenal metastases which contain little or none (Fig. 34). This relatively high lipid content of adrenal adenomas distinguishes them from other adrenal lesions. Using these criteria, an accuracy of 100% in the differentiation between adenoma and nonadenoma has been reported (Tsushima et al. 1993). These excellent results appear to directly reflect the simplicity of the technique employed. They are corroborated by two recent studies comparing the value of T2 relaxation times, tissue contrast enhancement characteristics, and chemical shift properties regarding differentiation of adrenal lesions (Korobkin et al. 1995; Reinig et al. 1994). Both studies confirmed the excellent accuracy of chemical shift imaging regarding the differentiation of adenomas from other nonadenomatous adrenal lesions. Phase-shift imaging does not permit differentiation among other etiologies including primary and secondary malignancies, pheochromocytoma, and inflammatory masses (Fig. 35).

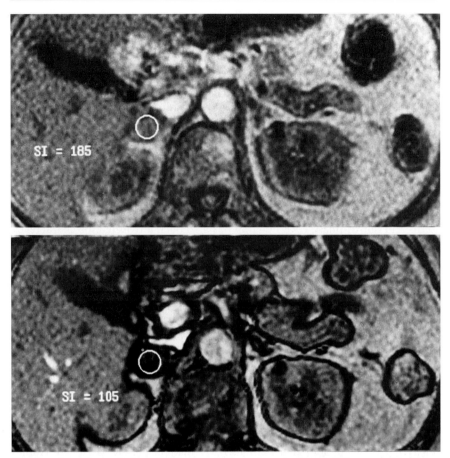

Fig. 33. In- and out-of-phase GRE images demonstrate a significant difference in SI within a region of interest placed over a 2 cm right adrenal mass. While the in-phase images were acquired with a TE of 4.6 ms, the out-of-phase images were acquired with a TE of 2.3 ms. The SI difference confirms the presence of intracellular fat and thus confirms the diagnosis of adrenal adenoma

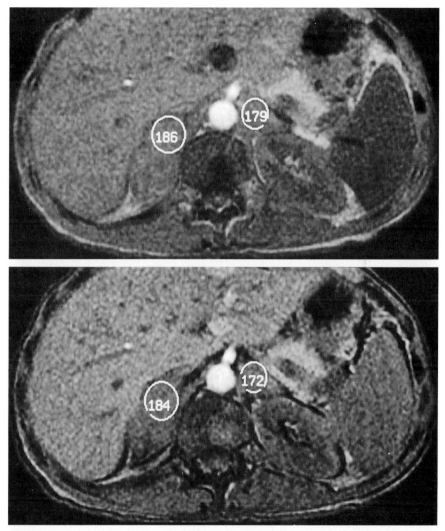

Fig. 34. Bilateral adrenal masses identified in a patient with bronchial carcinoma on in- and out-of-phase multiplanar GRE images. While the in-phase images were acquired with a TE of 4.6 ms, the out-of-phase images were acquired with a TE of 2.3 ms. Lack of a change in SI confirms the nonadenomatous nature of the masses. At biopsy bilateral metastases were confirmed

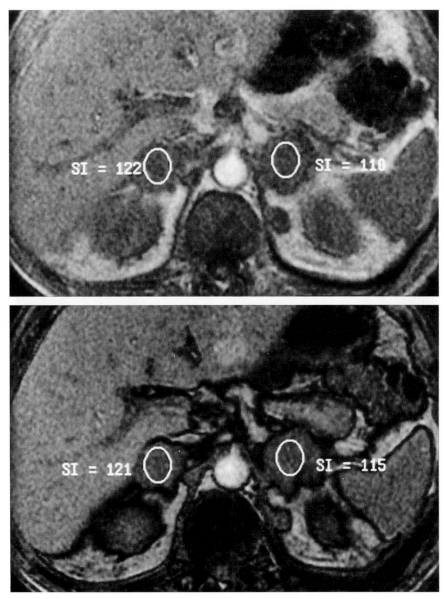

Fig. 35. Multiplanar GRE images acquired in- and out-of-phase identify bilateral adrenal masses. A lack of signal difference between the in- and out-of-phase images confirms the nonadenomatous nature of the lesions. In this case biopsy confirmed tuberculosis

4   Ultrafast 3D Gradient-Echo Imaging

In combination with the intravenous application of paramagnetic contrast agents, breath-held 3D spoiled GRE imaging has been shown to be useful in the depiction of arterial morphology. The technique permits a 3D display of vascular morphology and pathology. In many centers ultrafast contrast-enhanced 3D MR angiography has already become the modality of choice for evaluation of the thoracic aorta, abdominal aorta and its branches, and pelvic vasculature. Chapter 4 describes the potential of these exciting new applications in more detail.

The ultrafast 3D MR spoiled GRE technique can be adapted for depicting the stomach and colon. The 3D nature of the data acquisitions permits exploitation of a host of image postprocessing techniques, permitting analysis from both an "outer" (exoscopic) and an "inner" (endoscopic) perspective. The latter provides "virtual" endoscopic images. Hence it has become possible to render virtual colonoscopic and gastroscopic images.

4.1   MR Colonography

The latency of the polyp-based genesis of colonic cancer provides a lengthy screening window of 18–36 months during which simple polypectomy is curative (Murakami et al. 1990). As evidenced by the persistently high incidence of colonic cancer (Potter and Slattery 1993), this window is not taken advantage of for lack of a suitable screening modality (Lieberman 1994). A variety of tests have been evaluated for the detection of polyps. Serum tumor markers detect colonic cancer only in an advanced stage, while hemocult testing has been shown to be neither sensitive nor specific (Allison et al. 1996). Reflecting its projectional nature, double-contrast barium enema is characterized by limited sensitivity in the detection of polyps (Thoeni and Petras 1982). Higher sensitivities have been achieved with colonoscopy, which in most centers has become the modality of choice for evaluating of the colon (Lieberman and Smith 1991). In addition to considerable patient discomfort and difficulties in reaching the right colon, which has been shown to be increasingly predisposed to tumor development (Steele 1994), the relatively high costs associated with colonoscopy prevent its use for widespread screening (Lieberman 1991). Thus ultrafast 3D MR colonography may constitute an interesting diagnostic alternative.

Based on the principles of ultrafast contrast-enhanced 3D GRE acquisitions (Leung et al. 1996), breath-hold 3D colonography has become possible (Luboldt et al. 1997a; Figs. 36–39). For MR colonography the principles of contrast-enhanced 3D MR angiography are transferred from the arterial system to the colon. Instead of the arterial lumen, the colon is filled with T1-shortening paramagnetic contrast.

For MR colonography the patient is placed in a prone position onto the MRI table. Prior to the MR examination the patients' bowel is prepared in a manner similar to that required for conventional colonoscopy. The contrast enema is administered per rectum using a disposable enema kit with an inflatable tip (E-Z-EM, Westbury, NY, USA) by hydrostatic pressure (1–1.5 m water column) (Debatin et al. 1997). The enema consists of 1500–2000 ml water with 15–20 ml of a 0.5-mol Gd-DTPA solution (Magnevist; Schering, Berlin, Germany). To reduce bowel motion scopolamine (20 mg) is administered intravenously as the patient is placed on the MR table. Filling of the colon is monitored with a 2D non-slice-select acquisition, collecting one image every second. In addition to assuring adequate filling, this 2D overview allows recognition of both high-grade stenosis and peritoneal leakage (Debatin et al. 1997). Once the contrast agent has reached the cecum, 64 contiguous 2-mm sections of a 3D data set are acquired in a 28-s breath-hold (Potter and Slattery 1993). To enable differentiation of free-floating fecal material and air bubbles from fixed polypoid lesions the prone 3D acquisition is repeated following the intravenous administration of 0.1 mmol/kg Gd-DTPA. Finally, the patient is imaged in the supine position (Debatin et al. 1997).

Analysis of the MR colonographic data sets can be based on multiplanar reformation in addition to targeted maximum-intensity projections and virtual colonoscopic views (Fig. 36). Virtual colonoscopic images, displaying the inside of the colonic lumen can be constructed on a Sparc 20 Advantage Windows workstation (GE Medical Systems) using commercially available software (Navigator, GE Medical Systems). The diagnostic value of such virtual colonoscopic views was established in an in vitro study using ex vivo colonic specimen. Regarding the detection of polyps, virtual endoscopic viewing rendered vastly improved sensitivity and specificity values (87%/96%) compared to mere exoscopic inspection of the individual cross-sectional images alone (Schoenenberger et al. 1997; Figs. 37, 38).

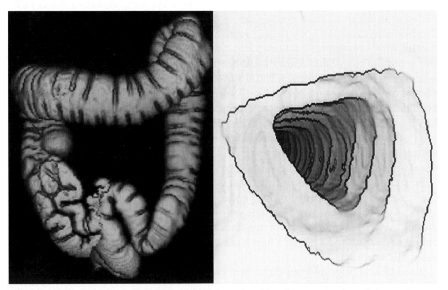

Fig. 36. *Left*, 3D surface-shaded display of the colon. The data set consists of 60 contiguous 2-mm sections acquired breath-held over 30 s, following colonic filling with an enema consisting of 2 l water with 20 ml Gd-DTPA. *Right*, virtual intraluminal endoscopy depicting the inside of the transverse colon (*arrows*) displays the haustral folds to good advantage

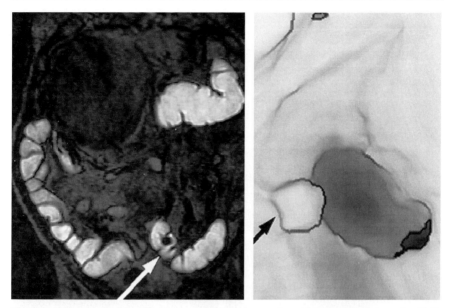

Fig. 37. Polyp of the sigmoid colon, 1 cm in size, seen on the multiplanar reconstruction (*left*) of a 3D MR colonographic data set and on the virtual colonoscopic image (*right*). The presence of the polyp was confirmed by conventional colonoscopy

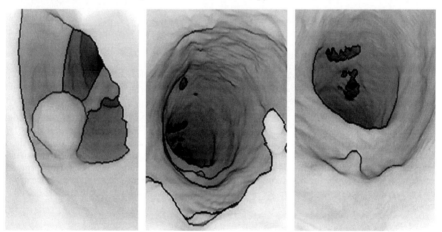

Fig. 38. MR colonography is capable of detecting polyps of various sizes. A 15-mm (*left*), 10-mm (*middle*), and even a sessile 6-mm (*right*) polyp were confidently diagnosed based on virtual colonoscopic images. Better spatial resolution will be required to detect polyps smaller than 5 mm

Initial in vivo experience is based on 21 patients who underwent both MR colonography and conventional colonoscopy within the same morning (Luboldt et al. 1997b). All subjects tolerated the 30-min MR colon examination well. MR colonography correctly assessed 9/11 mass-negative patients as negative and

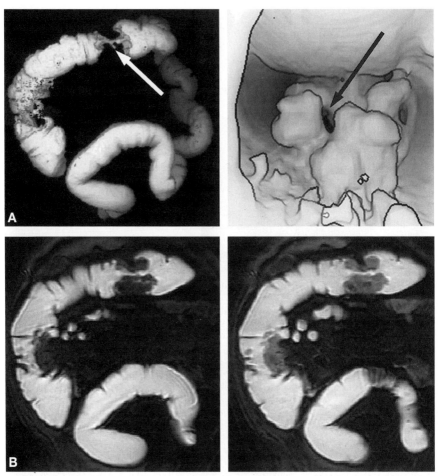

Fig. 39A, B. (A) Two colonic carcinomas in the transverse and ascending colon are identified on the 3D surface-shaded display projection (*left*). The lesion in the transverse colon is characterized by the pathognomonic apple core shape with a narrow channel (*arrow*). (B) Targeted maximum-intensity projections acquired before (*left*) and following (*right*) the administration of intravenous contrast show avid enhancement of the colonic mass lesions. Enhancement is confirmed in both lesions

6/10 mass-positive patients as positive. One of the missed positive patients (false negative) showed two polyps of 8 mm whereas the other three patients contained polyps smaller than 5 mm. No correlate (false positive) was found for three small polyps (5–10 mm), detected with MR colonography in two patients. The diagnostic performance of MR colonography depended on lesion size. All nine lesions exceeding 10 mm in size, and seven of ten masses measuring between 5 and 10 mm were correctly identified, while lesions smaller than 5 mm were not seen (Luboldt et al. 1997b). This inability to visualize small polyps is related directly to the large voxel size of up to 15 mm^3. Partial volume effects as well as smoothing algorithms in the employed software render these lesions invisible. Several strategies can be pursued to improve resolution. A further reduction in repetition time to below 2 ms (Wielopolski et al. 1997) allows acquisition of more MR data points within the same time frame. A different strategy involves use of zero-filling routines, in both the in-plane and the through-plane axis. These techniques are available today and result in a doubling of image resolution without lengthening scan time (Korosec et al. 1996).

Contrast enhancement following intravenous administration facilitated differentiation of polypoid masses from fecal material or air. In fact, enhancement could be demonstrated in all nine lesions larger than 10 mm and in four of the smaller polyps (Fig. 39). It may furthermore become of particular relevance in the evaluation of patients with inflammatory bowel disease. The administration of intravenous paramagnetic contrast also permits concomitant assessment of the liver. Unsuspected hepatic lesions were identified in two patients; both proved to be unsuspected liver metastases (Luboldt et al. 1997b).

The concept of 3D MR colonography illustrates how the combination of ultrafast 3D data-acquisition strategies coupled with novel postprocessing techniques opens a totally new application for MRI. Although conventional colonography is likely to remain the diagnostic standard of reference for the foreseeable future, MR colonography appears to have considerable potential with regard to colonic screening. Owing to the relatively short imaging times and limited amount of paramagnetic contrast required, the test could be offered at a reasonable cost. Lack of harmful side effects in conjunction with relative patient comfort during the examination promise to enhance patient acceptance. Clearly the potential of this technique to provide accurate, minimally invasive, cost-efficient polyp screening and comprehensive colonic tumor staging warrants further investigation.

4.2   MR Gastrography

Although upper gastrointestinal endoscopy is a safe and effective diagnostic procedure, complications do exist (Arrowsmith et al. 1991), and procedure-related costs are considerable (Gonvers et al. 1996). Furthermore, upper gastrointestinal endoscopy fails to recognize disease extension beyond the confines of the gastric wall, such as lymph node metastasis in the perigastric region. These limitations could be overcome by a noninvasive technique providing both endoscopic and exoscopic information.

Based on the principles of ultrafast, contrast-enhanced 3D GRE acquisitions (Leung et al. 1996), breath-hold 3D gastrography is possible. The subject is placed on the MR table in a left decubitus position with the head elevated. Blueberry juice is used as the base for the oral contrast. This contains manganese and hence causes considerable T_1-shortening (Hiraishi et al. 1995). To reduce the T_1 relaxation time even further, 2 ml of a gadolinium-chelate (Gd-DOTA, Dotarem, Guerbet Laboratories, Cedex, France) were added to the 400 ml contrast volume. Since only a small amount of paramagnetic contrast is required in addition to the blueberry juice, the contrast mix remains relatively inexpensive.

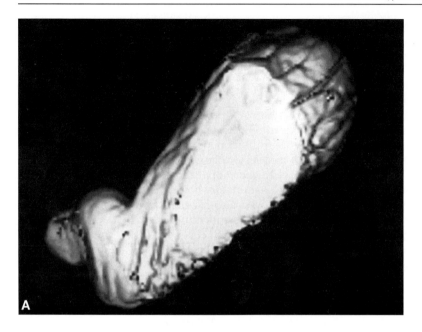

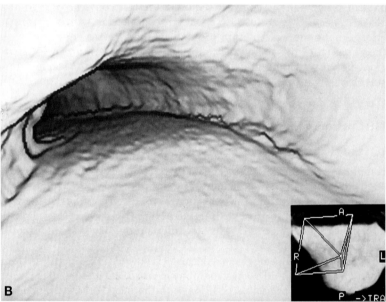

Fig. 40A, B. (A) Surface-shaded display image of a 3D data set depicting a normal stomach acquired in the 45° left lateral decubitus position. The stomach is homogeneously filled with contrast, which has not spilled beyond the duodenal bulb. The gastric folds are well appreciated. (B) Virtual intraluminal endoscopy of the gastric fundus details the regular gastric folds from an internal perspective. Limitations in spatial resolution are apparent

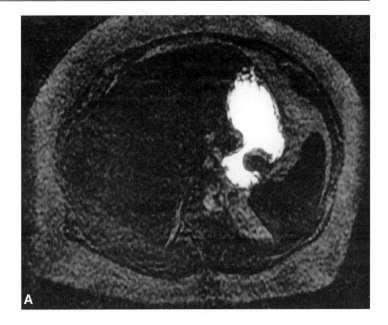

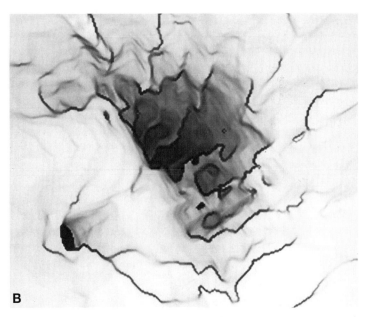

Fig. 41A, B. (A) Source image of a 3D gastric data set obtained in a patient (supine position) following gastric banding for morbid obesity. The stomach is filled with signalrich contrast. (B)Virtual intraluminal endoscopy of the proximal pouch permits assessment of the gastric folds and depicts the residual lumen following the banding procedure

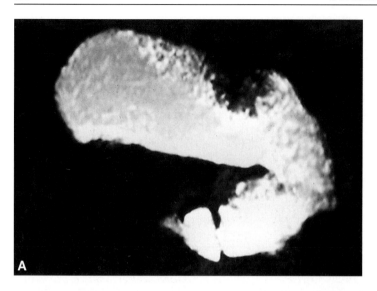

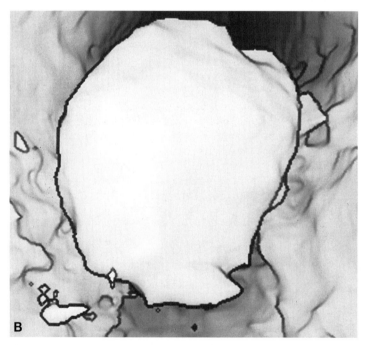

Fig. 42A, B. (A) Maximum-intensity projection image of the stomach in a patient with a polypoid gastric mass. The data were acquired breath-held in the supine position. The entire stomach and the duodenal bulb are filled with contrast. (B) Virtual intraluminal endoscopy of the gastric mass as seen from the fundus

Following ingestion of the contrast material the subject is advanced into the bore of the scanner. A 3D gradient-echo acquisition covering the stomach with 64 contiguous 2-mm sections is collected in 30 s (Figs. 40–42). To compensate for the presence of residual air in the stomach, the subject is imaged in the left lateral decubitus, supine, and finally right lateral decubitus position. Similarly as in MR colonography, the 3D data sets can be viewed in various manners (Figs. 40–42). Multiplanar reformations, providing an in depth understanding of gastric morphology, are available immediately following data acquisition. Volume calculations of the 3D data sets can provide virtual intraluminal endoscopic views of the stomach. The software is commercially available from GE Medical Systems. A full virtual gastroscopy consists of around 60 coned endoscopic views, the tip of which is located at the observer's position. The images are displayed with a frame rate of 10/s, and the resulting virtual gastroscopy is registered on video tape.

Early experience revealed MR gastrography to be well tolerated. Particularly the taste of the contrast agent was received enthusiastically. 3D MR gastrography provides a comprehensive endo- and exoscopic display of the stomach. Combined left lateral decubitus and supine data sets permit assessment of the entire stomach, from fundus to pylorus. The duodenal bulb is best visualized in the right lateral decubitus position. Analysis of the source images is helpful in patients with gastric banding (Fig. 41), where the interactive use of oblique multiplanar reformations allows the exact determination of the diameter of the residual lumen narrowed by the gastric band and in the evaluation of a large polypoid gastric mass (Fig. 42). For a true assessment of the mucosa better spatial resolution is clearly required. The implementation of zero-filling routines and the use of shorter repetition times will provide the tools for a further augmentation of spatial resolution in the forseeable future.

The combination of 3D gastric MRI with conventional forms of MRI enhances its utility. The use of contrast-enhanced, dynamically collected multiplanar acquisitions permit local, lymph node, and hepatic staging all within the same examination. Sequences exploiting the natural T1 and T2 contrast of the MR experiment may also be added as considered appropriate.

Undoubtedly, multiple aspects of gastric MRI will require improvements and further testing prior to a routine clinical implementation. It may well become another new application based upon the implementation of ultrafast 3D data-acquisition strategies.

5   Echo-planar Techniques

Echo-planar (EPI) data-acquisition strategies are capable of significantly shortening MRI times. The time resolution of EPI allows the acquisition of images in less than 100 ms, virtually eliminating motion-related artifacts. The high temporal resolution of EPI can be exploited to track moving organ systems in real time. Stehling et al. (1989) characterized the peristaltic pattern of the gastric antrum and proximal small intestine for fasting subjects before and following caloric stimulation. They demonstrated the feasibility of quantitating gastrointestinal tract motion with a single-shot EPI technique. In EPI data acquisitions temporal resolution is traded off against physical limitations regarding SNR and spatial resolution. These have to date prevented implementation of these techniques into routine clinical imaging protocols.

To improve spatial resolution several investigators have suggested using multishot EPI acquisitions. In contrast to single-shot EPI, the echo train is divided into several portions resulting in improved SNR, which can be used to enhance spatial resolution (McKinnon 1993; Butts et al. 1993) (Chapter 1). Using an eight-shot EPI strategy, breath-held T2-weighted echo-planar images of the liver were acquired with image quality comparable to that of conventional T2-weighted SE images (Butts et al. 1993). Reimer et al. (1992) have illustrated that SNR and hence spatial resolution can also be enhanced by using an inversion pulse. In their study single-shot T1-weighted EPI images of the pancreas acquired with an inversion time of 100 ms were characterized by a SNR similar to that of a two-shot SE EPI (Reimer et al. 1992). The overall resolution remained limited, however, with an in-plane resolution of 1.6 × 3.1 mm.

Goldberg et al. (1993) have used EPI data-acquisition strategies in conjunction with varying inversion times to increase the accuracy of T1 and T2 relaxation measurements of focal hepatic lesions. Considerable overlap of relaxivity values between various lesions limits the applicability of this technique, however. Finally, a most interesting application for EPI in the abdomen has been proposed by Müller et al. (1994). They used EPI to quantitate the molecular diffusion process in vivo throughout the abdomen. In vivo diffusion measurements were obtained in multiple abdominal organs of normal volunteers and a limited number of patients. The study revealed differences between the apparent diffusion coefficients of normal parenchymal tissue and that of lesions in the liver.

Despite these interesting works in progress the use of EPI in the abdomen cannot be recommended for routine clinical use at this time.

References

Aerts P, Van Hoe L, Bosmans H, Oyen R, Marchal G, Baert AL (1996) Breath-hold MR urography using the HASTE technique. AJR Am J Ronetgenol 166:543–545

Allison JE, Tekawa IS, Ransom LJ, Adrain AL (1996) A comparison of fecal occult blood tests for colorectal cancer screening. N Engl J Med 334 (3):155–159

Arrowsmith JB, Gerstmann BB, Fleischer DE et al (1991) Results from the American Society for Gastrointestinal Endoscopy/US Food and Drug Administration. Collaborative Study on complication rates and drug use during gastrointestinal endoscopy. Gastrointest Endosc 37:421–427

Bilbey JH, McLoughlin RF, Kurkjian PS, Wilkins GEL, Chan NHL, Schmidt N, Singer J (1995) MR imaging of adrenal masses: value of chemical-shift imaging for distinguishing adenomas from other tumors. AJR 164:637–642

Butts K, Riederer SJ, Ehman RL, Felmlee JP, Grimm RC (1993) Echo-planar imaging of the liver with a standard MR imaging system. Radiology 189:259–264

Catalano C, Pavone P, Laghi A et al (1996) Magnetic resonance pyelography: optimization of the technique and the preliminary results. Radiol Med Turino 91 (3):270–274

Constable RT, Smith RC, Gore JC (1992) Signal-to-noise and contrast in fast spin echo and inversion recovery FSE imaging. J Comput Assist Tomogr 16 (1):41–47

Davis CP, Ladd ME, Romanowski BJ, Wildermuth S, Knoplioch JF, Debatin JF (1996) Human aorta: preliminary results with virtual endoscopy based on three dimensional MR imaging data sets. Radiology 199:37–40

Debatin JF, Schoenenberger A, Bauerfeind P, Krestin GP (1997) In vivo exoscopic and endoscopic MR-imaging of the colon. American Journal of Radiology; in press

de Lange EE, Mugler JP, Bertolina J, Brookeman JR (1992) Selective versus nonselective preparation pulses in two-dimensional MR-RAGE MR imaging of the liver. JMRI 2:355–358

de Lange EE, Mugler III JP, Gay SB, DeAngelis GA, Berr SS, Harris EK (1996) Focal liver disease: comparison of breath-hold T1-weighted MP-GRE imaging and contrast-enhanced CT-lesion detection, localization, and characterization. Radiology 200:465–473

Di-Girolamo M, Pirillo S, Laghi A, Iannicelli E, Fini D, Amadei M, Pavone P, Passariello R (1996) Urography with magnetic resonance: a new method for the study of the renal collecting system in patients with obstructive uropathy. Radiol Med Torino 92 (6):758–764

Eilenberg SS, Lee JKT, Brown JJ, Mirowitz SS, Tartar VM (1990) Renal masses: evaluation with gradient-echo Gd-DTPA-enhanced dynamic MR imaging. Radiology 176:333–338

Gaa J, Hatabu H, Jenkins RL, Finn JP, Edelman RR (1996) Liver masses: replacement of conventional T2-weighted spin-echo MR imaging with breath-hold MR imaging. Radiology 200:459–464

Göhde SC, Toth J, Krestin GP, Debatin JF (1997) Dynamic contrast-enhanced multiplanar gradient-echo MR imaging of the pancreas: impact on diagnostic performance. Am J Radiol 68:689–696

Goldberg EM, Simunovic LM, Drake SL, Mueller WF Jr, Verrill HL (1989) Comparison of serum CA 19-9 and CEA levels in a population at high risk for colorectal cancer. Hybridoma 8 (5):569–575

Goldberg MA, Hahn PF, Saini S, Cohen MS, Reimer P, Brady TJ, Mueller PR (1993) Value of T1 and T2 relaxation times from echoplanar MR imaging in the characterization of focal hepatic lesions. AJR 160:1011–1017

Gonvers J-J, Burnand B, Froehlich F, Pache I, Thorens J, Fried M, Kosecoff J, Vader J-P, Brook RH (1996) Appropriateness and diagnostic yield of upper gastrointestinal endoscopy in an open-access endoscopy unit. Endoscopy 28:661–666

Hagspiel KD, Neidl KF, Hauser M, Duewell St, Marincek B (1994) Fettunterdrückte MR-Bildsequenzen in der Diagnostik von Neoplasien der Leber und des Pankreas bei 1,5 Tesla. RoFo 160:235–242

Hamed MM, Hamm B, Ibrahim ME, Taupitz M, Mahfouz AE (1992) Dynamic MR imaging of the abdomen with gadopentetate dimeglumine: normal enhancement patterns of the liver, spleen, stomach, and pancreas. AJR 158:303–307

Hamm B, Thoeni RF, Gould RG, Bernardino ME, Lüning M, Saini S, Mahfouz A-E, Taupitz M, Wolf K-J (1994) Focal liver lesions: characterization with nonenhanced and dynamic contrast material-enhanced MR Imaging. Radiology 190:417–423

Hiraishi K, Narabayashi I, Fujita O, Yamamoto K, Sagami A, Hisada Y, Saika Y, Adachi I, Hasegawa H (1995) Blueberry juice: preliminary evaluation as an oral contrast agent in gastrointestinal MR imaging. Radiology ;194:119-123.

Hirohashi S, Hirohashi R, Uchida H, Kitano S, Ono W, Ohishi H, Nakanishi S (1997) MR cholangiopancreatography and MR urography: improved enhancement with a negative oral contrast agent. Radiology 203 (1):281–285

Jung G, Krahe T, Kugel H, Gieseke J, Walter C, Fischbach R, Landwehr P (1996) Comparison of fast turbo-spin-echo and gradient- and spin-echo sequences as well as echo planar imaging with conventional soin-echo sequences in MRI of focal liver lesions at 1.0 tesla. Rofo Fortschr Geb Rontgenstr Neuen Bildgeb Verfahr 1996 35 (12):911–918

Kane AG, Redwine MD, Cossi AF (1993) Characterization of focal fatty change in the liver with a fat-enhanced inversion-recovery sequence. J Magn Reson Imaging 21 (1):82–83

Korobkin M, Lombardi TJ, Aisen AM, Francis IR, Quint LE, Dunnick NR, Londy F, Shapiro B, Gross MD, Thompson NW (1995) Characterization of adrenal masses with chemical shift and gadolinium-enhanced MR imaging. Radiology 197:411–418

Korosec FR, Frayne R, Grist TM, Mistretta CA (1996) Time-resolved contrast-enhanced 3D MR angiography. MRM 36:345–351

Kreft B, Layer G, Kuhl C, Sommer T, Gieseke J, Schild H (1995) Turbo spin echo sequences with selective fat supression (SPIR) in the MRI of focal liver lesions at 0.5 T. Rofo 163 (5):411–416

Kreft B, Steudel A, Textor J, Novak D, Muller B, Miersch WD, Schild H (1996) Magnetic reonance tomography of the kidney: the testing of new pulse sequences and comparison with CT in the differential diagnosis of space-occupying lesions. Rofo 164 (3):212–217

Laubenberger J, Büchert M, Schneider B, Blum U, Hennig J, Langer M (1995) Breath-hold projection magnetic resonance-cholangio-pancreatography (MRCP): a new method for the examination of the bile and pancreatic ducts. MRM 33:18–23

Leung DA, McKinnon GC, Davis CP, Pfammatter T, Krestin GP, Debatin JF (1996) Breath-hold, contrast-enhanced, three-dimensional MR angiography. Radiology 200 (2):569–571

Lieberman D (1991) Cost effectiveness of colon cancer screening. Am J Gastroenterol 86 (12):1789–1794

Lieberman D (1994) Colon cancer screening: beyond efficacy. Gastroenterology 106 (3):803–807

Lieberman DA, Smith FW (1991) Screening for colon malignancy with colonoscopy. Am J Gastroenterol 86 (8):946–951

Low RN, Francis IR, Sigeti JS, Foo TKF (1993a) Abdominal MR imaging: comparison of T2-weighted fast and conventional spin-echo, and contrast-enhanced fast multiplanar spoiled gradient-recalled imaging. Radiology 186:803–811

Low RN, Francis IR, Herfkens RJ, Jeffrey RB Jr, Glazer GM, Foo TKF, Shimakawa A, Pelc NJ (1993b) Fast multiplanar spoiled gradient-recalled imaging of the liver: pulse sequence optimization and comparison with spin-echo MR imaging. AJR 160:501–509

Low RN, Hinks RS, Alzate GD, Shimakawa A (1994) Fast spin echo MR imaging of the abdomen: contrast optimization and artifact reduction. J Magn Reson Imaging 4 (5):637–645

Low RN, Alzate GD, Shimakawa A (1997) Motion suppression in MR imaging of the liver: comparison of respiratory-triggered and nontriggered fast spin-echo sequences. AJR Am J Roentgenol 168 (1):225–231

Luboldt W, Bauerfeind P, Steiner P, Fried M, Krestin GP, Debatin JF (1997) Preliminary assessment of three-dimensional magnetic resonance imaging for various colonic disorders. Lancet 349:1288–1291

Luboldt W, SteinerP, Bauerfeind P, Pelkonen P, Debatin JF (1997b) Detection of Mass Lesions with MR-Colonography (MRC): Preliminary Report; Radilogy (in press)

Mathieu D, Rahmouni A, Anglade M-C, Falise B, Beges C, Gheung P, Mollet JJ, Vasile N (1991) Focal nodular hyperplasia of the liver: assessment with contrast-enhanced turboFLASH MR imaging. Radiology 180:25–30

McKinnon GC (1993) Ultrafast interleaved gradient-echo-planar imaging on a standard scanner. MRM 30:609–616

Megibow AJ, Zhou XH, Rotterdam H, Francis I, Zerhouni EA, Balfe DM, Weinreb JC, Aisen A, Kuhlmann J, Heiken JP, Gatsonis C, McNeil BJ (1995) Pancreatic adenocarcinoma: CT versus MR imaging in the evaluation of resectability – report of the Radiology Diagnostic Onocology Group. Radiology 195:327–332

Mitchell DG, Crovello M, Matteucci T, Petersen RO, Miettinen MM (1992a) Benign adrenocortical masses: diagnosis with chemical shift imaging. Radiology 185:345–351

Mitchell DG, Shapiro M, Schuricht A, Barbot D, Rosato F (1992b) Pancreatic disease: findings on state-of-the-art MR images. AJR 159:533–538

Mirowitz SA, Brown JJ, Lee JKT, Heiken JP (1991) Dynamic gadolinium-enhanced MR imaging of the spleen: normal enhancement patterns and evaluation of splenic lesions. Radiology 179:681–686

Müller MF, Pottumarthi P, Siewert B, Nissenbaum MA, Raptopoulos V, Edelman RR (1994) Abdominal diffusion mapping with use of a whole-body echo-planar system. Radiology 190:475–478

Murakami R, Tsukuma H, Kanamori S, Imanishi K, Otani T, Nakanishi K, Fujimoto I, Oshima A (1990) Natural history of colorectal polyps and the effect of polypectomy on occurrence of subsequent cancer. Int J Cancer 46 (2):159–164

Outwater EK, Siegelman ES (1996) MR imaging of pancreatic disorders. Magn Reson Imaging 8 (5):265–289

Outwater EK, Mitchell DG, Vinitski S (1994) Abdominal MR imaging: evaluation of a fast spin-echo sequence. Radiology 190:425–429

Pavone P, Catalano C, Cardone G et al (1995) Identification of pancreatic insulinomas. The role of magnetic resonance. Radiol Med Torino 90 (6):734–739

Peterson MS, Baron RL, Murakami T (1996) Hepatic malignancies: usefulness of acquisition of multiple arterial and portal venous phase images at dynamic gadolinium-enhanced MR imaging. Radiology 201:337–345

Potter JD, Slattery ML (1993) Colon cancer: a review of the epidemiology. Epidemiol Rev 15:499–545

Powell SM, Petersen GM, Krush AJ, Booker S, Jen J, Giardiello FM, Hamilton SR, Vogelstein B, Kinzler KW (1993) Molecular diagnosis of familial adenomatous polyposis. N Engl J Med 329 (27):1982–1987

Ramani M, Reinhold C, Semelka RC, Siegelman ES, Liang L, Ascher SM, Brown JJ, Eisen RN, Bret PM (1997) Splenic hemangiomas and hamartomas: MR imaging characteristics of 28 lesions. Radiology 202:166–172

Reimer P, Saini S, Hahn PF, Mueller PR, Brady TJ, Cohen MS (1992) Techniques for high-resolution echo-planar MR imaging of the pancreas. Radiology 182:175–179

Reinig JW, Stutley JE, Leonhardt CM, Spicer KM, Margolis M, Caldwell CB (1994) Differentiation of adrenal masses with MR imaging: comparison of techniques. Radiology 192:41–46

Rofsky NM, Weinreb JC, Bosniak MA, Libes RB, Birnbaum BA (1991) Renal lesion characterization with gadolinium-enhanced MR imaging: efficacy and safety in patients with renal insufficiency. Radiology 180:85–89

Rubin GD, Beaulieu CF, Argiro V, Ringl H, Norbash AM, Feller JF, Dake MD, Jeffrey RB, Napel S (1996) Perspective volume rendering of CT and MR images: applications for endoscopic imaging. Radiology 199:321–330

Saini S, Nelson RC (1995) Technique for MR imaging of the liver. Radiology 197:575–577

Schima W, Saini S, Echeverri JA, Hahn PF, Harisinghani M, Mueller PR (1997) Focal liver lesions: characterization with conventional spin-echo vesusu fast spin-echo T2-weighted MR imaging. Radiology 202:389–393

Schoenenberger A, Bauerfeind P, Krestin GP, Debatin JF (1997) Virtual colonoscopy with MRI: in vitro evaluation of a new concept. Gastroenterology 112:1863–1870

Schwartz LH, Seltzer SE, Tempany SM et al (1993) Prospective comparison of T2-weighted fast spin-echo, with and without fat suppression, and conventional spin-echo pulse sequences in the upper abdomen. Radiology 189 (2):411–416

Semelka RC, Simm FC, Recht M, Deimling M, Lenz G, Laub GA (1991) T1-weighted sequences for mr imaging of the liver: comparison of three techniques for single-breath, whole-volume acquisition at 1.0 and 1.5 T. Radiology 180:629–635

Semelka RC, Shoenut JP, Kroeker MA, Greenberg HM, Simm FC, Minuk GY, Kroeker RM, Micflikier AB (1992a) Focal liver disease: comparison of dynamic contrast-enhanced CT and T2-weighted Fat-suppressed, FLASH, and dynamic gadolinium-enhanced MR imaging at 1.5 T. Radiology 184:687–694

Semelka RC, Shoenut JP, Kroeker MA, MacMahon RG, Greenberg HM (1992b) Renal lesions: controlled comparison between CT and 1.5-T MR imaging with nonenhanced and gadolinium-enhanced fat-suppressed spin-echo and breath-hold FLASH techniques. Radiology 182:425–430

Semelka RC, Cumming MJ, Shoenut JP, Magro CM, Yaffe CS, Kroeker MA, Greenberg HM (1993a) Islet cell tumors: comparison of dynamic contrast-enhanced CT and MR imaging with dynamic gadolinium enhancement and fat suppression. Radiology 186:799–802

Semelka RC, Shoenut JP, Magro CM, Kroeker MA, MacMahon R, Greenberg HM (1993b) Renal cancer staging: comparison of contrast-enhanced ct and gadolinium-enhanced fat-suppressed spin-echo and gradient-echo MR imaging. JMRI 3:597–602

Semelka RC, Brown ED, Ascher SM, Patt RH, Bagley AS, Li W, Edelman RR, Shoenut JP, Brown JJ (1994) Hepatic hemangiomas: a multi-institutional study of appearance on T2-weighted and serial gadolinium-enhanced gradient-echo MR images. Radiology 192:401–406

Sittek H, Heuck AF, Fölsing C, Gieseke J, Reiser M (1995) Statische und dynamische Kernspintomographie des Pankreas: Kontrastmittelkinetik des normalen Pankreasparenchyms bei Pankreaskarzinomen und chronischer Pankreatitis. Fortschr Rontgenstr 162:396–403

Steele GD Jr (1994) The National Cancer Data Base report on colorectal cancer. Cancer 74(7):1979–1789

Stehling MK, Evans DF, Lamont G, Ordidge RJ, Howseman AM, Chapman B, Coxon R, Mansfield P, Hardcastle JD, Coupland RE (1989) Gastrointestinal tract: dynamic MR studies with echo-planar imaging. Radiology 171:41–46

Taupitz M; Hamm B; Speidel A; Deimling M; Branding G; Wolf KJ (1992) Multisection FLASH: method for breath-hold MR imaging of the entire liver. Radiology 183: 73-9

Thoeni RF, Petras A (1982) Double-contrast barium-enema examination and endoscopy in the detection of polypoid lesions in the cecum and ascending colon. Radiology 144:257–260

Tsushima Y, Ishizaka H, Matsumoto M (1993) Adrenal masses: differentiation with chemical shift, fast low-angle shot MR imaging. Radiology 186:705–709

Van Hoe L, Bosmans H, Aerts P, Baert AL, Fevery J, Kiefer B, Marchal G (1996) Focal liver lesions: fast T2-weighted MR imaging with half-Fourier rapid acquisition with relaxation enhancement. Radiology 201:817–823

Wallner BK, Schumacher KA, Weidenmaier W, Friedrich JM (1991) Dilated biliary tract: evaluation with MR cholangiography with a T2-weighted contrast-enhanced fast sequence. Radiology 181:805–808

Wernecke K, Rummeny E, Bongartz G, Vassallo P, Kivelitz D, Wiesmann W, Peters PE, Reers B, Reiser M, Pircher W (1991) Detection of hepatic masses in patients with carcinoma: comparative sensitivities of sonography, CT, and MR imaging. AJR 157:731–739

Whitney WS, Herfkens RJ, Jeffrey RB, McDonnell CH, Li KCP, Van Dalsem WJ, Low RN, Francis IR, Debatin JF, Glazer GM (1993) Dynamic breath-hold multiplanar spoiled gradient-recalled MR imaging with gadolinium enhancement for differentiating hepatic hemangiomas from malignancies at 1.5 T. Radiology 189:863–870

Wielopolski PA, Hicks, de Bruin H, Oudkerk M (1997) Localizing pulmonary emboli: combining breathhold three-dimensional lung perfusion imaging and 512 matrix pulmonary angiography after contrast administration. Book of abstracts ISMRM 1997

Yamashita Y, Mitsukaki K, Yi T, Ogata I, Nishiharu TN, Urata J, Takahashi M (1996) Small hepatocellular carcinoma in patients with chronic liver damage: prospective comparison of detection with dynamic MR imaging and helical CT of the whole liver. Radiology 200:79–84

Zerhouni EA, Rutter C, Hamilton SR, Balfe DM, Megibow AJ, Francis IR, Moss AA, Heiken JP, Tempany CMC, Aisen AM, Weinreb JC, Gatsonis C, McNeil BJ (1996) CT and MR imaging in the staging of colorectal carcinoma: report of the Radiology Diagnostic Oncology Group II. Radiology 200:443–451

Subject Index

Printing: Druckhaus Beltz, Hemsbach
Binding: Buchbinderei Schäffer, Grünstadt